THE SIRTFOOD DIET COOKBOOK

THE SIRTFOOD DIET COOKBOOK: WHY SIRT RECIPES ARE THE REVOLUTION IN DIETING. 101 SIRTFOOD DIET RECIPES FOR BEGINNERS THAT LET YOU DRINK WINE EAT CHOCOLATE AND GET THE BODY YOU HAVE ALWAYS DREAMED OF

BEATRICE MORELLI

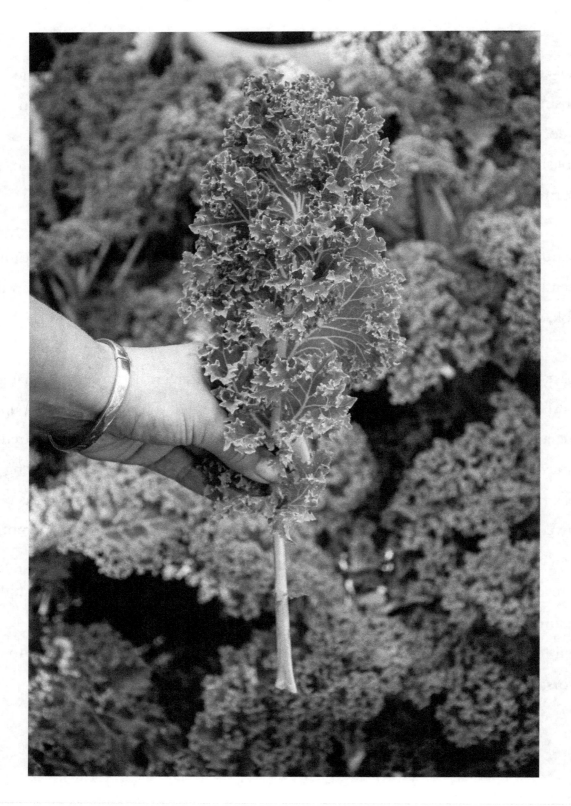

TABLE OF CONTENTS

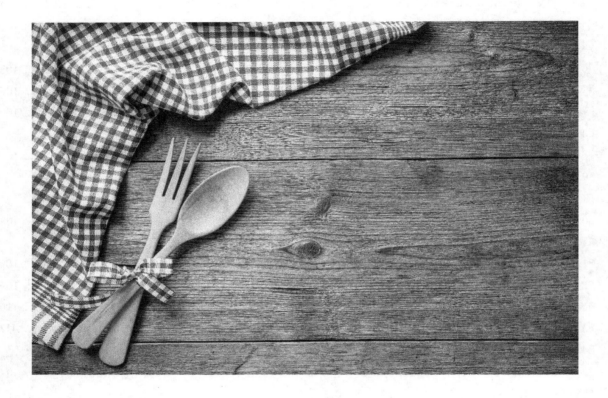

Introduction

The Sirtfood diet attempts to emulate the advantages of fasting diets, but without any of the drawbacks. You will learn about the theory of fasting diets and how the Sirtfood diet cleverly achieves the same effect, but without any of the actual fasting's.

Many fasting diets have become popular over the past five years. The most well-known are the several variants of the intermittent fasting structure, such as the five-two diet. In the five-two food, you fast during the weekend and usually eat during the working days of the week. These diets have proven and demonstrated effects on longevity, weight loss and overall health.

That is because these fasting diets activate the 'skinny gene' in our body. This gene causes the fat-storage processes to shut down and for the body to enter a state of 'survival' mode, which in turn causes the body to burn fat.

Burning fat is what you might expect if you necessarily start starving yourself. Still, another interesting effect of fasting is that your body switches from the replication of cells to the repair of cells.

Anytime cells in your body replicate, there is a small chance of your D.N.A. damaged in the process. However, if your body repairs dying and older cells, there is no risk of D.N.A. damage, which is the reason why fasting is associated with a lower prevalence of the degenerative disease, such as Alzheimer's.

However, the problem with fasting diets, as the name implies, is that you have to fast. Fasting feels awful, mainly when we surrounded by other people having regular eating habits. It also puts some social spotlight on your diet – explaining to your co-workers or your extended family why you are not eating on certain days is bound to generate wonder and challenges to your diet regime.

Furthermore, even though fasting has numerous associated benefits, there are some downsides too. Fasting is associated with muscle loss, as the body doesn't discriminate between muscle mass and fat tissue when choosing cells to burn for energy.

Fasting also risks malnutrition, only by not eating enough foods to get essential nutrients. This risk can be somewhat alleviated by taking vitamin supplements and eating nutrient-rich foods. Still, fasting can also slow and halt the digestive system altogether – preventing the absorption of supplements. These supplements also need dietary fat to be dissolved, which you might also lack if you were to implement a strict fasting method.

On top of this, fasting isn't appropriate for a massive range of people. You don't want children to fast and potentially inhibit their growth. Likewise, the elderly, the ill, and the pregnant are all just too vulnerable to the risks of fasting.

Additionally, there are several psychological detriments to fasting, despite commonly being associated with spiritual revelations. Fasting makes you irritable and causes you to feel slightly on edge – your body is telling you always that you need to forage for food, enacting physical processes that affect your mood and emotions.

That is why the authors of the Sirtfood diet sought a replacement for fasting diets. Fasting is beneficial for our body, but it just isn't practical for society at large. That is where sirtuin activators and Sirtfoods come to the rescue.

Sirtuins first discovered in 1984 in yeast molecules. Of course, once it became apparent that sirtuin activators affected a variety of factors, such as lifespan and metabolic activity, interest in these proteins blossomed.

Sirtuin activators boost your mitochondria's activity, the part of the biological cell which is responsible for the production of energy. That, in turn, mirrors the energy-boosting effects, which also occur due to exercise and fasting. The Sirt food diet is hard to start a process called adipogenesis, which prevents fat cells from duplicating – which should interest any potential dieter.

The exciting part is that sirtuin activators influence your genetics. The notion of the 'genetic' lottery embedded in the public consciousness, but genes are more changeable then you might think. You won't be able to change your eye color or your height, but you can activate or deactivate specific genes based on environmental factors. That is called epigenetics, and it is a fascinating field of study.

Sirtuin activators cause the S.I.R. genes to activate, the before-mentioned 'skinny genes', which in turn increases the released. Sirts or Silent Information Regulators also help regulate the circadian rhythm, which is your natural body clock and influences sleep patterns.

Sleep is essential for many vital biological processes, including those that help regulate blood sugar (which is also crucial for losing weight). If you find yourself always stuck in a state of lag and brain fog, this may cause by your circadian rhythm is out of sync, which is another way the Sirt food diet can help your body.

Additionally, Sirts help contains free radicals. Free radicals are not as impressive as the sound – they are A.W.O.L. particles in your body that damage your D.N.A. and speed up the ageing process.

To summaries, the Sirtfood diet contains foods, which are high in sirtuin activators. Sirtuin activators activate your S.I.R. genes or 'skinny genes' which enact beneficial metabolic processes. These processes, which involve molecules, called Sirts, cause your body to burn fat, repair human cells and combat free radicals.

Evidence

So, sirtfoods have hailed as the next dietary wonder – but where is the cold, hard evidence? Well, the proof of the Sirt food diet comes from multiple sources. To start with, Aidan Goggins and Glen Matten, the originators of the Sirtfood diet, performed their trial at a privately owned fitness Centre to test sirtfoods themselves.

At a fitness Centre called K.X., in Chelsea, London, the two authors of the Sirt food diet selected their clientele eat a carefully monitored constructed Sirt food diet. What is particularly interesting about the study is that weight wasn't the only variable measured – the researchers also measured body composition and metabolic activity – they were searching for the holistic effect of the diet.

97.5% of people managed to stick to the first-three day fasting period, involving only 1000 calories. Generally speaking, this is a much higher rate of success than typical fasting diets, where many people have their willpower shattered in just the first few days.

Out of the 40 participants, 39 completed the study. In terms of overall fitness and weight, the individuals in the education were well distributed – 2 were officially obese, 15 fell into the overweight category while 22 had a natural body mass index. There were also 21 women and 18 men – a diet for both the genders! However, with that said, being members of a fitness Centre, the individuals in the study were more likely to exercise more than the standard population – a potential confounding factor.

Participants lost over 7lbs on average in the first week. Every participant experienced an improvement in body composition, even if their gains were not as dramatic as their peers.

There were also numerous reported psychological benefits, although these were not formally quantified. These improvements include an overall sense of feeling and looking better. As a side note, it also claimed the 40 participants rarely felt hungry, even despite the calorie deficits imposed by the diet.

The most startling result from the Sirt food diet is that muscle mass after the 1-week diet period was either the same as before or showed slight improvements. Dieting law typically states that when losing fat, muscle is also lost, usually around 20-30% of the total weight loss, you should lose 2-3 lbs. of muscle for every 10 pounds lost.

Of course, retaining muscle isn't just better from an overall fitness perspective, but also a beautiful view. A common fear, especially in men, is that if they lose weight is that they will look skinny, scrawny, and unhealthy. Yet by the retaining the muscle you will gain that toned, slither look that is so fashionable in models.

Another essential reason why retaining muscle mass is your resting energy expenditure. Your muscles require energy, even when you are not using them intensely. Owing to this, people who keep skeletal muscle burn more calories than people who don't, also if both people are sedentary. Being muscular allows you to eat more calories and get away with it!

Muscle mass has also associated with a general decrease in degenerative diseases as you age (such as diabetes and osteoporosis) as well as lower rates of mental health problems (such as depression and excessive anger).

Overall, the clinical trial performed at the K.X. Fitness Centre not only supported the notion that the Sirtfood diet can aid weight loss and promote holistic body health, but it also leads to the surprising finding that sirtfoods can retain muscle mass.

Blue Zones

The other evidence for the power of Sirtfoods comes from the 'blue zones'. The blue zones are small regions in the world where people miraculously live longer than everywhere else.

Perhaps most startlingly, you don't just see people live longer in blue zones; you still see them retain energy, vigor, and overall health even in their advanced years. Most of us have a fear of becoming frail, immobile, and overall miserable as we age.

Furthermore, we envision this as starting to occur in our forties and fifties, while becoming a fixed reality in our sixties, seventies, and eighties. Yet in the blue zones, people not only live past 100 surprisingly regularly but can walk, work and exercise just as well as those in the younger years. Likewise, they remain mentally slide and don't suffer the cognitive deficits we typically associate with old age.

The blue zones include several areas of the Mediterranean, Japan, Italy, and Costa Rica. What do these regions all have in common? They all eat a diet high in sirtfoods. The Mediterranean is famous for its healthy diet involving copious amounts of fish and olive oil. The Japanese savor matcha green tea, while the Costa Ricans traditionally indulge in cocoa, coffee and more.

That is the beauty of the Sirt food diet – it isn't trying to make your eating habits artificial and awkward. It is merely copying the healthiest practices that already exist around the world.

Chapter 1:

The Science Behind Sirtuins

The Sirt food diet can't classify as low-carb or low-fat. This diet is quite different from its many precursors while advocating many of the same things: the ingestion of fresh, plant-based foods. As the name implies, this is a sirtuin based diet, but what are sirtuins and why have you never heard about them before?

There are seven sirtuin proteins – SIRT-1 to SIRT-71. They can find throughout your cells and the cells of every animal on the planet. Sirtuins are found in almost every living organism and practically every part of the cell, controlling what goes on. Supplement company, Elysium Health, likens the body's cells to an office with sirtuins acting as the CEO, helping the cells react to internal and external changes. They govern what done when done, and who does is.

Of the seven sirtuins, one works in your cell's cytoplasm, three in the cell's mitochondria, and another three in the cell's nucleus. They have a full number of jobs to perform, but mostly they remove acetyl groups from other proteins. These acetyl groups signal that the protein they are attached to is available to perform its function. Sirtuins remove the available flag and get the protein ready to use.

Sirtuins sound pretty crucial to your body's normal function, so why is that you've never heard of them before?

The first sirtuin to be discovered was SIR2, a gene found in the 1970s which controlled the ability of fruit flies to mate. It wasn't until the 1990s that scientists discovered other, similar proteins, in almost every form of life. Every organism had a different number of sirtuins – bacteria has one and yeast has five. Experiments on mice show they have the same amount as humans, seven.

Sirtuins have shown to prolong life in yeast and mice. There is, so far, no evidence of the same effect in human beings. However, these sirtuins are present in almost every form of life, and many scientists are hopeful that if organisms as far apart as yeast and mice can see the same effect from sirtuin activation, this may also extend to humans.

In addition to sirtuins, our bodies need another substance supplement for cells to function correctly. Elysium (see above) likens this substance to the money a company needs to keep operating. Like any CEO, a sirtuin can only keep the company working correctly if the cash flow is sufficient. NAD+ first discovered in 1906. You get your supply of NAD+ from your diet by eating foods made up the building blocks of NAD+.

Fun Facts about Sirtuins:

1. Mice that have engineered to have high levels of SIRT-1 are both more active and leaner than average, while mice that lack SIRT-1 altogether are fatter and more prone to various metabolic conditions.

2. Add the fact that levels of SIRT-1 are much lower in obese people than in those of a "healthy" weight, and the case for the importance of sirtuins in weight loss becomes compelling.

3. By making a permanent change to your diet and adding the best sirtfoods to your eating plan, the authors of the Sirt food diet believe everyone can achieve better health, all without losing muscle mass.

To Sum Up

Exercise and calorie restriction are both sources of stress which encourage our bodies to adapt to changing circumstances. If the pressure becomes too high, the result can be an injury, the body can even die, but at lower levels, we adapt, and this temporary, low-level stress is key to many physiological changes.

For example, stress on muscles, enough but not too much, is what makes the body increase muscle mass.

Similarly, the authors of the Sirt food diet found that it is when the body is stressed, by exercise or low-calorie intake, that the effect of sirtuins kicks in and it is this effect that can be reproduced by a diet rich in SIRT foods.

Is this the diet for you?

Any diet plan you adopt involves some level of expense and inconvenience. It may also involve risk. Anyone can write a diet book, as there is no need to have the diet medically approved. That's one reason why all foods start by suggesting you consult a doctor. One thing you can do is look at the qualifications of the diet's author.

The authors of the Sirt food diet are not TV personalities or reality stars. They have genuine scientific knowledge of the subject, and both have master's degrees to prove it.

Aidan Goggins is a pharmacist, with a degree in pharmacy and a master's degree in Nutritional Medicine. Glen Matten trained at the Institute for Optimum Nutrition before completing his master's degree in nutritional medicine.

The Sirt food diet is not their first collaboration. In 2012, they wrote, "The Health Delusion," a book that attacked many of the "long-held truths" of the diet and health industry. As a result, they received the consumer health book of the year award by the Medical Journalists Association.

Having reviewed the literature and asked the big question: "What would happen if we ate sirtfoods? Would there be weight loss?" they went on to ask: "What would happen to muscle mass, which usually lost during almost any diet?"

To find the answers, the authors conducted a trial in an exclusive health spa near London in the UK. There were 40 participants. Thirty-nine completed the test. Because the experiment carried out at a health spa, the authors had complete control over the food eaten by the participants. Note that this is not always the case in "medical" trials where the participants report what they ate.

The discovery and history of sirtuins

There were different quantities of sirtuins in every creature. For instance, yeast has five sirtuins, microscopic organisms have one, mice have seven, and people have seven.

The way that sirtuins found across species imply they were "saved" with development. Qualities that are "rationed" have all-inclusive capacities in numerous or all species. What was at this point to be known, however, was how significant sirtuins would end up being.

In 1991, Elysium fellow benefactor and MIT scholar Leonard Guarente, nearby alumni understudies Nick Austriaco and Brian Kennedy, led trials to all the more likely see how yeast matured. By some coincidence, Austriaco attempted to develop societies of different yeast strains from tests he had put away in his ice chest for quite a long time, which made a distressing domain for the tensions. Just a portion of these strains could develop from here, yet Guarente and his group identified an example: The pressures of yeast that endure the best in the cooler were likewise the longest-lived. That gave direction to Guarente so he could concentrate exclusively on these long-living strains of yeast.

That prompted the identification of SIR2 as a quality that advanced life span in yeast. It's critical to note more research required on SIR2's belongings in people. The Guarantee lab consequently found that expelling SIR2 abbreviated yeast life range significantly. In particular, expanding the number of duplicates of the SIR2 quality from one to two grew the life length in yeast. In any case, what initiated SIR2 usually presently couldn't seem to be found.

That is the place acetyl bunches become possibly the most crucial factor. It was at the first idea that SIR2 might be a deacetylating protein — which means it expelled those acetyl gatherings — from different atoms. Yet, nobody knew if this were valid since all endeavors to show this movement in a test tube demonstrated negative. Guarantee and his group had the option to find that SIR2 in yeast could supply different proteins within sight of the supplements.

In Guarantee's own words: "Without NAD+, SIR2 sits idle. That was the basic finding on the circular segment of sirtuin science."

Chapter 2:

Top 20 Sirtfoods

- Arugula
- Buckwheat
- Capers
- Celery
- Chilies (birds' eye chilly)
- Cocoa (pure or in 85% chocolate)
- Coffee
- Dates (Medjoul)
- Green tea
- Kale
- Lovage
- Olive oil
- Onions (red)
- Parsley
- Radicchio
- Red wine
- Soya
- Strawberries
- Turmeric
- Walnuts

The following 40 other sirtuin-activating foods also recommended in the Sirt food diet. These are not quite as strongly activating as those from the top 20 list but are still highly recommended.

Fruits

apples · blackberries · cranberries · goji berries · raspberries · currants (black) · kumquats · plums · grapes (red)

Vegetables and legumes

artichokes · broccoli · watercress · chicory (light) · broad beans · white beans · green beans · last salad · bok choy · shallots · asparagus · onions (white)

Beverages

black tea · white tea

Cereals

popcorn · quinoa · whole meal flour

Herbs and spices

chilly · dill · ginger · mint · oregano · legend · chives · thyme

Nuts and seeds

chia seeds · peanuts · chestnuts · pecan nuts · pistachios · sunflower seeds

How can it work?

At its Centre, the way to getting in shape is fundamental: create a calorie shortage either by expanding your calorie consume exercises or diminishing your caloric admission. Be that as it may, imagine a scenario where you could avoid the dieting and rather actuate a "thin quality" without the requirement for extraordinary calorie limitation. That is the reason for the Sirt food diet, composed by nourishment specialists Aidan Goggins and Glen Matten. The best approach to do it, they contend, is sirtfoods.

Sirtfoods are wealthy in supplements that enact a purported "thin quality" called sirtuin. As indicated by Goggins and Matten, the "thin quality" acted when a lack of vitality made after you confine calories. Sirtuins got intriguing to the sustenance world in 2003 when scientists found that resveratrol, a compound found in red wine, had a similar impact on life length as calorie limitation yet it was accomplished without decreasing admission. (Discover the absolute truth about wine and its medical advantages.)

In the 2015 pilot study (led by Goggins and Matten) testing the adequacy of sirtuins, the 39 members lost a normal of seven pounds in seven days. Those outcomes sound unbelievable, yet it's imperative to understand this is a small example size concentrated over a brief timeframe. Weight-loss specialists additionally have their questions about the elevated guarantees. "The cases made are theoretical and extrapolate from considers which generally centered around straightforward creatures (like yeast) at the cell level. What occurs at the cell level doesn't mean what occurs in the human body at the large-scale level," says Adrienne Youdim, m.d., the chief of the Centre for Weight Loss and Nutrition in Beverly Hills, CA. (Here, look at the best and most exceedingly awful diets to follow this year.)

The food executed in two stages. Stage one endures three days and limits calories to 1,000 every day, comprising of three green juices and one sirtfood-endorsed supper. Step two keeps going four days and raises the everyday designation to 1,500 calories for each day with two green juices and two dinners.

After these stages, there is an upkeep plan that isn't centered around calories yet instead on reasonable bits, well-adjusted suppers, and topping off on principally sirtfoods. The 14-day upkeep plan highlights three dinners, one green juice, and a couple of sirtfood chomp snacks. Adherents additionally urged to finish 30 minutes of movement five days per week-per government proposals; however, it isn't the fundamental focal point of the arrangement.

What are the advantages?

You will get thinner if you follow this diet intently. "Regardless of whether you're eating 1,000 calories of tacos, 1,000 calories of kale, or 1,000 calories of snickerdoodles, you will get in shape at 1,000 calories!" says dr. Youdim. In any case, she additionally calls attention to that you can have accomplishment with an increasingly sensible calorie limitation. "The run of the mill every day caloric admission of somebody not on a diet is 2,000 to 2,200, so lessening to 1,500 is as yet limiting and would be a powerful weight-loss procedure for most," she says.

Chapter 3:

The Sirtfood Diet

S tarting the Sirtfood diet is very easy. It just takes a bit of preparation. If you do not know what Kale is, or where you would find Green Tea, then you may have a learning curve, albeit very small. There is little in the way of starting the Sirtfood diet.

Since you will be preparing and cooking healthy foods, you may want to do a few things the week you start:

1. Clear your cabinets and refrigerator of foods that are unhealthy, and that might tempt you. You also will have a very low-calorie intake at the start, and you do not want to entice into a quick fix that may set you back. Even though you will have new recipes, you may feel that your old comfort foods are more comfortable at the moment.

2. Go shopping for all of the ingredients that you will need for the week. If you buy what you will need, it is more cost-effective. Also, once you see the recipes, you will notice that many ingredients overlap. You will get to know your portions as you proceed with the diet, but at least you will have what you need and save yourself some trips to the store.

3. Wash, dry, cut and store all of the foods that you need that way you have them conveniently prepared when you need them. That will make a new diet seem less tedious.

One necessary kitchen tool that you will need aside from the real foods is a juicer. You will need a juicer as soon as you start the Sirtfood diet. Juicers are everywhere, so they are quite easy to find, but the quality ranges greatly, however. That is where price, function, and convenience come into play. You could go to a famous department store, or you can find them online. Once you know what you are going after, you can shop around.

The quality of the juicer will also determine the nutritional quality and sometimes the taste of your juice, which we will explain. Just know that buying a cheap juicer may seem like a good idea now, but if you decide to upgrade, you will have spent more money, and twice. If you buy a good juicer, think of it as an investment in your health. Many people have paid cash for a gym membership that went unused for quadruple the cost of one juicer. A juicer won't go to waste.

So, since not all juicers are alike, let us list a few of the features that you want to look.

Centrifugal juicers:

Centrifugal juicers do just that, and they use centrifugal force to spin the food (most like vegetables like carrots, cucumbers, or kale leaves) at high speeds to the sidewalls, where there are blades. The food pushed through a sieve, and then you have your juice. You have to drink this rather quickly, as you will lose nutrients the longer it exposed to air (which it already has done as it was spinning), and it oxidizes, as well as a bit of heat from the friction which creates a loss of nutrients and enzymes. That is the whole reason you are juicing, so this point is quite essential. You also left with a lot of solid but very wet pulp as a byproduct, which also means there was a lot of fibrous parts of the plants that the juicer couldn't handle. That is also a missed opportunity for more nutrients. You will also get a lot of (warmish) foam at the top, which some people do not like. It is quick, and it is easy, however, and it is usually the cheapest of the juicer types. If you must, it is better than not having one at all, but if you can invest, you will reap your rewards later.

Masticating juicers:

Masticating juicers also do what they say they are. They masticate or chew the food, albeit more slowly than the other type, by pulling it through gears, which extract the juice. The machine pushes the pulp out. You would have less flesh with this machine afterwards. There is also less oxidation, and thus, more nutrients. They also can handle other types of foods (which vary by make and model), but that is something you should consider. You will get some foam with this as well, but not as much. These are more expensive, and again, should be looked at as you would an investment that you would not use and toss away. If you want it to last, and you want to get the most from your juicing and take it seriously, you will want to spend a bit more money and get what you need.

Twin-gear/triturating juicers:

These geared juicers have geared that grind together with millimeters of space left between, to tear open foods and grind the plants with only a dehydrated pulp that is left. These are the most nutrient-efficient juicers on the market. They leave virtually no foam, and they are nutrient-dense as they are not disturbing the inner plant cells with oxidation. You usually can tell in the look (color) and taste (more productive) than other juices. You can use different attachments to make different foods with most brands as well, so they are versatile. This highest pricing of most juicers in general, and there are also brand variations as with the others.

Citrus Juicers

There are also juicers specifically for citrus fruits. These can range from handheld, col-press juicers, to small electric or automatic cold-press juicers. They too vary in quality and price,

You can do a bit of research on the juicers that you may need. It will help engage you're more in the process and the journey you are about to take!

Storing Juices

The most nutrition from them immediately, you should drink them right away. If needed, you can pre-juice, and put these in glass jelly, Mason jars. The wide mouth variety with the plastic lids is tasty, airtight, and non-corrosive.

You can chill your drinks for the day, by resting them on ice packs in an insulated lunch tote or cooler. In extreme cases, you could juice one to three days of them (it is recommended at the maximum for optimal freshness, although you could push it further out.

You may also find something to keep the juice chilled even while you are drinking at home. You can put a jar in the refrigerator just before prepping, and after your sauce, pour it into one. You can make it a regular ritual of sorts. Have "your glass" that you get ready every day. If you prefer straws, you can even buy yourself a pleasant, reusable glass straw. None of these things is necessary for the diet, but any juice just tastes so much better when it is not from plastic.

Here are some other tips to help you get started:

Drink your juices as the earlier meals in the day if it helps you. It is a great way to start your day for three reasons.

• It will give you energy for breakfast and lunch especially. By not having to digest dense foods, your body saves time and energy usually spent on moving things around to go through all the problematic motions. You will be guaranteed to feel lighter and more energetic this way. You can always change this pattern after the maintenance phase, but you may find that you want to keep that schedule.

• Having fruits and vegetables before starchy or cooked meals, no matter how healthy the ingredients, is the best way to go for your digestion. Fruits and vegetables digest more rapidly, and the breakdown into the compounds that we can use more readily. Think of it as having your salad before your dinner. It works in the same way. The more substantial foods, grains, oils, meats, etc., take more time to digest. If you eat these first, they will slow things down, and that is where you have a backup of food needing to break down. That is also when you may find yourself with indigestion.

• Juices, especially green juices, contain phytochemicals that not only serve as antioxidants, but they contribute to our energy and mood. You will notice that you feel much differently after drinking a green juice than you would if you had eggs and sausage. You may want to make a food diary and note things such as this!

Be prepared to adjust to having lighter breakfasts for a little while. Most often, we fill up with high protein, carbohydrate, and high-calorie meals early in the day. We may feel that we did not get enough to eat and that we are not full at first. Oddly as it sounds, we may even miss the action of chewing. Some people need to chew their food to feel like they have had a filling meal. It is something automatic that we do not think. Some also will miss that crunch such as with toast. Just pay attention to this, and know this is normal, and that it will pass.

Activation of sirtuins

Although our understanding of the exact functions of all the Sirtuins is minimal, studies show that activating them can have the following benefits:

Switching on fat burning and protection from weight gain: Sirtuins do this by increasing the functionality of the mitochondrion (which is involved in the production of energy) and sparking a change in your metabolism to break down more fat cells.

They were improving memory by protecting neurons from damage. Sirtuins also boost learning skills and mind through the enhancement of synaptic plasticity. Synaptic plasticity refers to the ability of synapses, weaken or strengthen with time due to a decrease or increase in their activity. That is important because memories represented by different interconnect network of synapses in the brain and synaptic plasticity is an essential neurochemical foundation of memory and learning.

Slowing down the Ageing Process: Sirtuins act as cell guarding enzymes. Thus, they protect the cells and slow down their aging process.

Repairing cells: The Sirtuins repair cells damaged by re-activating cell functionality.

Protection against diabetes: this happens through prevention against insulin resistance. Sirtuins do this by controlling blood sugar levels because this diet calls for moderate consumption of carbohydrates. These foods cause increases in blood sugar levels; hence the need to release insulin, and as the blood sugar levels increase significantly, there is a need to produce more insulin. Over time, cells become resistant to insulin; hence, the need to produce more insulin, and this leads to insulin resistance.

Fighting Cancers: The chemicals working as sirtuin activators affect the function of sirtuin in different cells, i.e. by switching it on when in healthy cells and shutting it down in cancerous cells. That encourages the death of cancerous cells.

Fighting inflammation: Sirtuins have a powerful antioxidant effect that has the power to reduce oxidative stress. That has positive effects on heart health and cardiovascular protection.

Chapter 4:

How To Follow The Sirtfood Diet

The Sirtfood Diet split into two stages spanning three weeks. After that, you should start "serve" your diet by consuming as many Sirt foods as practicable. The essential recipes of these have two phases contained in the Sirtfood Diet book, published by the makers of this diet. You will need to buy it to adopt the diet plan.

The meals have lots of sirtfoods, however, do include other components besides merely the "top 20 sirtfoods."

The majority of the sirtfoods and components are simple to discover.

Three of the signature ingredients needed for these two stages-- matcha green tea lovage, powder, and buckwheat-- might be costly or challenging to discover.

Phase 1: 7lb in Seven Days

The first phase lasts seven days and includes calorie limitation and lots of green juice. It intended to jump-start your weight reduction and declared to assist you to lose 7 pounds (3.2 kg) in seven days.

Throughout the very first three days of stage one, calorie consumption restricted to 1,000 calories. You consume three green juices in a day plus one sirtfood meal.

Types of meals include miso-glazed tofu, the sirtfood omelet, or buckwheat deep-fry shrimp.

On days 4-- 7 of stage one, calorie consumption increased to 1,500. That consists of two green juices in a day and two more Sirt food-rich meals, which you can select from the book.

Stage Two.

Phase two lasts for two weeks. Throughout this "maintenance" stage, you must continue to lose weight steadily.

There is no particular calorie limit for this phase. Instead, you eat three meals complete of sirtfoods and one green juice each day.

After the Diet.

You might duplicate these two stages as typically as wanted for more weight reduction.

After these stages, you are encouraged to continue "helping" your diet plans by including Sirt food in your meals regularly.

There is a range of Sirtfood Diet books which contain plenty of Sirt foods.

You can likewise include sirtfoods in your diet as a treat or in dishes you already utilize.

Additionally, you are motivated to continue drinking green juice every day.

In this method, the Sirtfood Diet ends up being more of a way of life modification than a one-time diet.

Lifestyle Advice

The Sirtfood diet was an achievement nourishment system a couple of years and was the dear eating routine with the broadsheet press at the time. If you missed it, the features are that it incorporates red wine, chocolate, and espresso. Far less promoted and eye-catching, (yet similarly uplifting news as we would like to think) is the way that the response to the inquiry, 'would you be able to eat meat on the Sirt nourishment diet?', is a resonating, yes.

The eating routine arrangement not just incorporates a decent sound part of the meat; it proceeds to recommend that protein is a fundamental consideration in a Sirtfood-based eating routine to receive the greatest reward.

We're not supporting this as some meat overwhelming eating routine (we despite everything recollect the awful breath from Atkins), it's in reality very veggie-lover cordial. It provides food for practically everybody, which is the thing that makes it so reasonable an alternative to us.

So, what is the Sirtfood diet? It was created by nutritionists Aidan Goggins and Glen Matten, following a pilot learn at the elite XK Gym, (Daniel Craig, Madonna and an entire host of different celebs are supposedly individuals) where they are the two experts in Sloane Square, London. Members in the preliminary lost 7lbs in the initial seven days, in what the creators call the hyper-achievement to organize. The science behind Sirtfoods drops out of an investigation in 2003 which found that a compound found in red wine, expanded the life expectancy of yeast. At last, this prompted the studies which clarify the medical advantages of red wine, and how (whenever drank reasonably) individuals who drink red wine put on less weight.

A significant part of the science behind Sirtfood diet is like 'fasting-diets' which have well known for as far as barely any years, where our bodies initiate qualities and our fat stockpiling turned off. Our bodies change to endurance mode, thus weight reduction. The negatives to fasting-eats fewer cars are the unavoidable craving that results, alongside a decrease in vitality, bad-tempered conduct (when you're "hangry"), weariness and muscle misfortune. The Sirtfood diet professes to counter those negatives, as it's anything but a quick. Hence, hunger isn't an issue, making it ideal for individuals who need to lead a functioning, reliable way of life.

Sirtfoods are a (generally newfound) gathering of nourishments that are incredible in actuating the 'sirtuin' qualities in our body, which are the qualities enacted in fasting eats fewer carbs. Leucine is an amino corrosive found in protein, which praises and upgrades the activities of Sirtfoods. That implies the ideal approach to eat Sirtfoods is by consolidating them with a chicken bosom, steak, or another wellspring of leucine, for example, fish or eggs.

Generally, we can thoroughly observe the advantage and intrigue of the Sirtfood diet. Like practically any eating regimen plan, it tends to be a faff getting every one of the fixings, and the 'Sirtfood green juice', which shapes a centerpiece of the initial 14 days of the arrangement, is a torment to make and costly. Yet, it shows improvement over you'd anticipate. We just trialed a couple of days of the method and keeping in mind that there was perceptible weight reduction, the genuine advantage of the book is the reasonable methodology of bringing Sirtfoods into your regular dinner arranging.

Wellbeing

"A few people say that the heart is the organ with which we think and that it feels torment and uneasiness. Yet, it isn't so. Men should realize that from the cerebrum, and the mind just emerges our delights, delights, chuckling, and tears. Through it, specifically, we think, see, hear, and recognize the appalling from the excellent, the terrible from the great, and the lovely from the disagreeable. To cognizance, the cerebrum is emissary" Hippocrates.

"The issue of nervous system science is to comprehend man himself," said the neurocartographer Dr More out of control Penfield. By and by, I wonder whether the human mind can ever accomplish comprehension of its complicated procedure? In such a manner, Tom Wolfe once said that the cerebrum being limited, and hard wired, it will most likely never have the ability to grasp human presence in any total manner.

Be that as it may, with the coming of the 'cerebroscope' and 'imaging neuroscience,' the 'backwoods' of the mind can't be rejected as just a "bowl of curds" as once scorned by logician Henry More. The neuroscientists show up as the envoys of another time, the 'Neurocentric Age', ready to explain the last puzzles of humanity in clarifying insight and neural working, the reproduction of the working cerebrum territory through huge jumps in innovation. I might want to emphasize that the Neurocentric age is the period wherein the cerebrum is focal not exclusively to the body yet to our origination of us. Neuroessentialism sets that, in every way that matters, we are our cerebrums. The advancement of man and progress identified with the development of the human mind has now made ready for the eurocentric world.

During a time where we remain as far as mental wellbeing and cerebrum sound way of life to save the social and psychological capital of the world? In perspective on the 'human maturing time bomb,' a 'pandemic of our century,' have we outlined a change in attitude in our general wellbeing approaches for 'Cerebrum solid way of life 2020?' Have we imagined the coming decade to be the 'Time of Brain Fitness?' Have we considered the effect of way of life infections time bomb, the Achilles impact point of modernization, coming about because of actualization, Coca-Cola colonization, inexpensive food, and Mc Donalization in our Indian culture?

Despite what might expect an examination by Joosten, and partners distributed in American Heart Association diary, Stroke 2013 underscored that cardiovascular wellbeing, cerebrum wellbeing, and cognizance are interlaced. Having a 'World Heart Day,' it is grievous to watch a complete disregard on cerebrum wellbeing mindfulness.

A reminder for critical changes in our Indian national wellbeing arrangements would be fundamental in the wake of taking cognizance of the discoveries of an examination by the Kessler Foundation Research Center, US and SreeChitraTirunal Institute for Medical Sciences and Technology, India, in 2012.

This investigation uncovered a shrouded plague of neurological incapacities moving through India coming from clutters, for example, dementia, stroke, and horrendous cerebrum wounds. In India, 27% of the populace is beneath destitution level. This way, the monetary weight of way of life issue in India is probably going to be excessively experienced by poor people.

Phase 2: Maintenance

Congratulations! You have finished the first "hardcore" week. The second phase is more comfortable and is the actual incorporation of sirtuin-filled food selections to your everyday diet or meals. You can call this the "maintenance stage".

By doing so, your body will undergo the fat-burning stage and muscle gain plus a boost on your immune system and overall health.

For this phase, you can now have three balanced SirtFood-filled meals each day plus one green juice a day.

There is no "dieting", but more on choosing healthier alternatives with adding SirtFood in each meal as much as possible.

I will be providing some recipes for tasty dishes with SirtFood inclusion to give you further an idea on how exciting and healthy this diet journey is.

Now you move back up to a regular calorie intake intending to keep your weight loss steady and your Sirtfood intake high. You should have experienced some degree of weight loss by now, but you should also feel trimmer and re-invigorated.

Chapter 5:

Questions and Answers

1 - Should the Sirtfood diet be associated with physical activity?

Physical activity alone is not enough to lose weight. But those who follow the Sirt diet should perform moderate physical activity for thirty minutes five times a week because it is beneficial for health and stimulates the activation of sirtuins.

2 - Does taking foods rich in protein and polyphenols make this diet safer than the others?

People should be encouraged to follow a diet rich in polyphenols. We know that they bring many health benefits, including increasing the mechanisms that regulate longevity and reducing the risk of cardiovascular disease. That makes it a positive diet if you don't think you can sustain this type of food for long periods.

3 — Can everyone does it?

There is no universal diet that is suitable for anyone; at the base, there is always the hormonal functioning, metabolism, sex, age, pathological states, habits, tastes to be kept in mind. However, it is not suitable for children and adolescents, underweight people and in the presence of nutritional deficiencies or eating disorders.

4 — Can athletes also eat the Sirt diet?

Yes. Indeed, Sirt foods have become a winning strategy for many sports champions, allowing them to achieve the goals set in terms of body composition and, more generally, of fitness.

5— Is it suitable for obese people?

Yes. Based on studies on the activity of sirtuins, they can derive the maximum benefits not only from losing weight but also in terms of general well-being. Obesity increases the risk of suffering from chronic diseases, the same from which Sirt foods help you protect yourself.

6 — Is it possible to lose fat but not muscle tone?

Yes, the slimming type of the Sirt diet is just that. In any other diet, if someone loses 3.5 kg per week, at least 900 grams are of muscle. Sirt foods, on the other hand, activate not only fat consumption, but also promote muscle growth and repair. That means that not only do you lose weight, but you also have a better and more toned appearance.

7 — Can I eat all the Sirt foods I want, even the high-calorie ones, and lose weight anyway?

Yup! Thanks to the effects on metabolism and appetite, you don't have to worry about eating too many Sirt foods. We do not invite you to binge, but to eat these foods until you feel satisfied. The only exception dates. In terms of drinks, the consumption of red wine must be, but this is obvious to everyone, responsible.

8 — What are the possible side effects?

The side effects exist even though the Sirt diet characterized by a large variety of healthy and beneficial foods for our body. It is easy to fall back on:

• nutritional deficiencies (iron, proteins, calcium, sugar) • tiredness • fatigue • mood swings
• excessive weight loss • headache • difficulty concentrating • pressure drops

Furthermore, taking too many quantities of centrifuges, therefore of liquids, can alter the metabolism causing nausea and intestinal problems. But these are affecting that people who are discouraged from dieting can manifest, as we have already said, that is, to children and adolescents, underweight people, in convalescence and the presence of nutritional deficiencies or eating disorders. Generally, a healthy person does not experience any side effects.

9 — Is it true that it promotes longevity?

Yes, in a certain sense, sirtuins are miracles of nature, because they regulate the metabolism of our body. And yes, it is scientifically proven that in the cultures where more Sirt foods ate the incidence of cancer is lower. Heart disease, diabetes, dementia, and osteoporosis are just some of the conditions that can prevent by activating sirtuins.

10 — Who is it recommended?

The Sirt diet is not suitable for everyone, this regime is recommended if you try to lose a few pounds quickly, but not if the slimming you want provides for a more substantial loss and a duration in time. However, this type of diet does not have significant contraindications, but only if followed in the times and in the ways provided without prolonging the times that require a limited calorie intake.

—For whom is it not recommended?

Even the Sirt diet can become harmful because it still provides foods that can be harmful to people with gastritis, colitis, nickel allergy, reflux. Of course, any diet deserves the advice of your doctor before starting it.

9 — What about the few calories ingested? In this diet, carbohydrates reduced, and fewer calories to take. Still, by increasing the consumption of foods capable of activating sirtuins, they make this food program balanced because it provides all the necessary nutrients.

Chapter 6:

Recipes

The Sirt Diet includes specific foods, and we would like to show some recipes to make at home. Some methods to prepare, after consulting with your doctor who will be able to evaluate your health and the most suitable diet, to make you lose weight in total safety.

1. **Chicken with Red Onion and Black Cabbage**

Preparation time: 0 mins

Cooking time: 35 mins

Servings: 3

Ingredients:

0.27 lb of chicken breast

0.28 lb of tomatoes

One chili pepper

One tablespoon of capers

0.18 oz of parsley

Lemon juice

2 tbsp. Extra virgin olive oil

Two teaspoons of turmeric

1.8 oz of cabbage

0.7 oz of red onion

One teaspoon fresh ginger

1.8 oz of buckwheat

Directions:

Marinate the chicken breast for 10 minutes with 1/4 of lemon juice, one tablespoon of extra virgin olive oil and one teaspoon of turmeric powder. Cut 0.28 lb of chopped tomatoes, remove the inside, season with Bird's Eye pepper, one tablespoon of capers, one teaspoon of turmeric and one of extra virgin olive oil, 1/4 of lemon juice and 0.18 oz of parsley chopped. Fry the chicken breast, dripped from the marinade, on a high flame for one minute on each side, then put it in the oven for about 10 minutes at 220 ° C. Let it rest covered with aluminum foil. Steam the chopped kale for 5 minutes.

Sauté red onion, a teaspoon of grated fresh ginger and a teaspoon of extra virgin olive oil; add the cooked cabbage and cook for a minute on the fire. Boil the buckwheat with a teaspoon of turmeric, drain, and serve with chicken, tomatoes, and chopped cabbage.

Nutrition:

Calories: 100 Cal Fat: 1 g

Fiber: 0 Carbs: 10 g Protein: 2 g

2. Turkey with Cauliflower CousCous

Preparation time: 0 mins

Cooking time: 35 mins

Servings: 2

Ingredients:

0.33 lb of turkey

5.3 oz of cauliflower

1.4 oz of red onion

One teaspoon fresh ginger

One bird's eye pepper

One clove of garlic

Three tablespoons of extra virgin olive oil

Two teaspoons of turmeric

1 oz of dried tomatoes

0.36 oz of parsley

Dried sage to taste

One tablespoon of capers

1/4 of fresh lemon juice

Directions:

Blend the raw cauliflower tops and cook them in a teaspoon of extra virgin olive oil, garlic, red onion, chili pepper, ginger, and a teaspoon of turmeric.

Leave to flavor for a minute, then add the chopped sun-dried tomatoes and 0.18 oz of parsley over the heat. Season the turkey slice with a teaspoon of extra virgin olive oil, the dried sage and cook it in another teaspoon of extra virgin olive oil. Once ready, season with a tablespoon of capers, 1/4 of lemon juice, 0.18 oz of parsley, a tablespoon of water and add the cauliflower.

Tips

Chocolate*

Choose dark chocolate with 85% cocoa, rich in antioxidants, and it has a low glycemic index.

Green tea**

Known because it is so good for our body, green tea contributes to the loss of fat, preserving the muscles. Choose the Matcha variety and drink it with the addition of a little lemon juice, which increases the absorption of the nourishing activators of sirtuins.

Chili pepper***

To spice up your dishes, use Bird's Eye (also called Thai) chili pepper, which is very rich in sirtuins.

You can use it at least three times a week.

Coffee

You can drink 3-4 cups a day being careful not to overdo it with sugar and avoid adding milk.

Nutrition:

Calories: 394 Cal Fat: 20 g Fiber: 8
Carbs: 28 g Protein: 28 g

3. Buckwheat Salad

Preparation time: 15 mins

Cooking time: 25 mins

Servings: 4

Ingredients:

5.3 oz of buckwheat

5.3 oz of frozen beans (or fresh if in season)

One courgetti

One carrot

One clove of garlic

0.7 oz of salted capers

One handful of sesame seeds (or sunflower)

Some basil leaves

One teaspoon hot pepper

One teaspoon balsamic vinegar to taste

Extra virgin olive oil to taste

Salt to taste.

Directions:

First, blanch the beans in abundant salted water until they cooked but al dente. Peel and cut the carrot into cubes half a centimeter thick. Do the same with courgetti. Cook the vegetables.

In a non-stick pan, heat a drizzle of extra virgin olive oil with the garlic clove. As soon as it has taken a little color and flavored the oil, remove it, and add the chopped carrots. Cook for about 5 minutes, then add the courgettis and cook on a high flame for another 10 minutes, being careful not to burn the vegetables. A few minutes after the end of cooking, add the broad beans and season with the chili pepper, capers, sesame seeds and coarsely chopped basil by hand. Stir to mix all the ingredients well and season with salt. Cook the wheat. Boil the buckwheat in abundant salted water, then drain it al dente and season it with the vegetables. Add the balsamic vinegar and mix before serving. Buckwheat salad can keep in an airtight container and the refrigerator for a couple of days.

Nutrition:

Calories: 388 Cal

Fat: 3 g

Fiber: 2 g

Carbs: 80 g

Protein: 7 g

4. Farro with Vegetables and Chicken
Preparation time: 45 mins
Cooking time: 45 mins
Servings: 2
Ingredients:
11.3 oz of spelled,

2 courgettis,

3 carrots,

2 potatoes,

5.3 oz of green beans,

5.3 oz of peas,

0.67 lbs of chicken,

1 onion,

2 cloves of garlic,

Extra virgin olive oil,

Parsley,

Salt to taste.

Directions:

Wash the spelled and cook it in boiling salted water for 25 minutes. Wash and cut the vegetables. In a pan, brown the onion and the garlic cloves minced in 3 tablespoons of oil, add the diced chicken, brown it, sprinkle with a little white wine, let it evaporate, add one ladle of broth, salt to taste and cook for 20 minutes. At this point, add the vegetables and continue cooking for 10 minutes. Drain the spelled and add it to the chicken and vegetables. Mix and cook for a few minutes over low heat, add chopped parsley and serve.

Nutrition:

Calories: 340 Cal Fat: 16 g

Fiber: 0 g Carbs: 33 g Protein: 15 g

5. Vegetable Soup

Preparation time: 0 mins

Cooking time: 55 mins

Servings: 2

Ingredients:

Carrots 0.18 lb Red onions 0.18 lb

White courgettis 0.33 lb Potatoes 0.73 lb

Salt to taste Black pepper to taste

Celery 0.13 lb Auburn tomatoes 0.77 lb

Borlotti beans 0.44 lb

Clean pumpkin 0.55 lb

Extra virgin olive oil 0.11 lb

Leeks 0.33 lb

Clean cauliflower 0.66 lb

Peas 0.44 lb

Rosemary 1 sprig

Laurel 2 leaves

Water to taste

Directions:

The vegetable soup starts by washing and drying the vegetables. Then take the pumpkin and remove the outer skin with a knife with a large blade. Remove the seeds and internal filaments with the help of a spoon. Then cut it into slices of equal thickness and then into cubes of about 0.4 inches on the side. Wash and peel the courgettis, cut them into slices, and cut them into cubes. Then shell the beans, then from the latter cut into cubes. Proceed with the tomatoes: remove the stalk and cut them into slices. Then also reduce the vegetables into cubes. Also finely chop celery. To finish, tie the sprigs of rosemary with bay leaves to create an aromatic bunch. Now all the ingredients for preparing the vegetable minestrone are ready. Pour the oil into a large pot with lid carrots, celery, onion, and leek and brown gently for about ten minutes, stirring often. Once the sautéed vegetables softened add the fragrant bunch and pour the beans. Cover with water: it will have to cover the vegetables by an inch. Wait for the boiling point and cook for 2 minutes. Add the pumpkin and repeat the same procedure: add water until it covers by an inch, wait for the boil to resume, and cook for 2 minutes. Same thing with the potatoes, and to follow with the cauliflower. Cover with more water put the lid and cook 25 minutes from the resumption of the boil. After 25 minutes add courgettis, peas and tomatoes, add water if necessary, season with salt and pepper and cook again 2-3 minutes after boiling still.

Nutrition:

Calories: 80 Cal Fat: 0 g

Fiber: 16 g Carbs: 0 g Protein: 3 g

Chapter 7:

Breakfasts

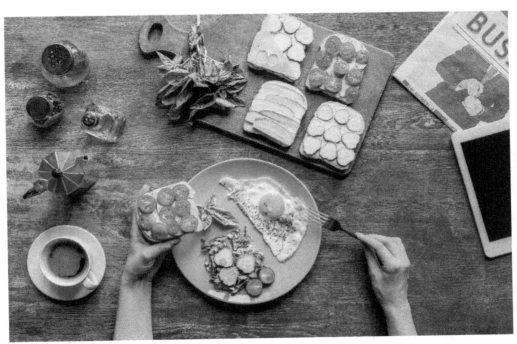

6. Sirtfood Mushroom Scrambled Eggs

Preparation time: 0

Cooking time: 10 mins

Servings: 2

Ingredients:

2 tbsp

1 teaspoon ground garlic

1 teaspoon mild curry powder

0.7 oz lettuce, approximately sliced

1 teaspoon extra virgin olive oil

1/2 bird's eye peeled, thinly chopped

A couple of mushrooms, finely chopped

0.18 oz parsley, finely chopped

Optional - insert a seed mix for a topper plus some rooster sauce for taste

Directions:

Mix the curry and garlic powder and then add just a little water until you've achieved a light glue. Steam the lettuce for 2 - 3 minutes. Heat the oil in a skillet over a moderate heat and fry the chili and mushrooms 2-3 minutes until they've begun to soften and brown. Insert the eggs and spice paste and cook over a moderate heat then add the carrot and then proceed to cook over a moderate heat for a further minute. In the end, put in the parsley, mix well, and serve.

Nutrition:

Calories: 182 Cal Fat: 12g

Fiber: 0 Carbs: 4g Protein: 12g

7. Turkey Breakfast Sausages

Preparation time: 20 mins

Cooking time: 3 -4 mins

Servings: 5

Ingredients:

1 lb. extra lean ground turkey

1 tbsp EVOO 9 Extra Virgin Olive Oil), and a little more to coat pan

1 tbsp fennel seeds

2 teaspoons smoked paprika

1 teaspoon red pepper flakes

1 teaspoon peppermint

1 teaspoon chicken seasoning

A couple of shredded cheddar cheese

A couple of chives, finely chopped

A few shakes garlic and onion powder

Two spins of pepper and salt

Directions:

Preheat oven to 350 F. Utilize a little EVOO to grease a miniature muffin pan. Combine all ingredients and blend thoroughly. Fill each pit on top of the pan and then cook for approximately 15-20 minutes. Each toaster differs therefore when muffin temperature is 165 then remove.

Nutrition:

Calories: 41 Cal Fat: 1.91g

Fiber: 0 Carbs: 0g Protein: 5.53g

8. Morning Meal Sausage Gravy

Preparation time: 20 mins

Cooking time: 10 -12 mins

Servings: 10

Ingredients:

1 lb. sausage

2 cups 2% milk (whole milk is great also)

1/4 cup whole wheat flour

Salt and a lot of pepper to flavor

Directions:

Cook sausage from skillet. Add flour and blend cook for about a minute. Insert two cups of milk.

Whisk whilst gravy thickens and bubbles. Add pepper and salt and to taste until perfect. Let stand a minute or so to scrape it over desired foods.

Nutrition:

Calories: 347 Cal

Fat: 26.47 g Fiber: 0.2 g

Carbs: 16.87 g Protein: 16.68 g

9. Easy Egg-White Muffins

Preparation time: 35 mins

Cooking time: 20 mins

Servings: 3

Ingredients:

English muffin - I enjoy Ezekiel 7 grain

Egg-whites - 6 tbsp or two large egg whites

Turkey bacon or bacon sausage

Sharp cheddar cheese or gouda

Organic berry

Optional- lettuce, and hot sauce, hummus, flaxseeds, etc...

Directions:

Get a microwavable safe container, then spray entirely to stop the egg from adhering, then pour egg whites into the dish. Lay turkey bacon or bacon sausage paper towel and then cook.

Subsequently, toast your muffin, if preferred. Then put the egg dish in the microwave for 30 minutes. Afterward, with a spoon or fork, then immediately flip egg within the dish and

cook for another 30 minutes. Whilst the dish remains hot, sprinkle some cheese while preparing sausage. The secret is to get a paste of some kind between each coating to put up the sandwich together, i.e. - a very small little bit of hummus or even cheese.

Nutrition:

Calories: 17 Cal Protein: 3.6 g

Fat: 0.06 g Fiber: 0 g Carbs: 0.24 g

10. Asparagus Mushroom Artichoke Strata

Preparation time: 0

Cooking time: 50 mins

Servings: 10

Ingredients:

1 small loaf of sourdough bread

4 challah rolls

8 eggs

2 cups of milk

1 teaspoon salt

1/4 teaspoon black pepper

1 cup fontina cheese, cut into little chunks

1/2 cup shredded parmesan cheese

1 tbsp butter (I used jojoba)

1 teaspoon dried mustard

1/2 can of artichoke hearts, sliced

1 bunch green onions, grated

1 bunch asparagus, cut into 1-inch bits

1 10oz package of baby Bella (cremini) mushrooms, chopped

Directions:

Clean mushrooms and slice and trim asparagus and cut in 1-inch pieces. Place in a bowl and scatter 1/2 teaspoon salt mixture. Drain and dice 1/2 can or medium artichoke hearts. Melt butter in a pan over medium heat, also sauté the asparagus and mushrooms before the mushrooms start to brown. Do this for about 10 minutes. Blend the artichoke core pieces into a bowl with all a mushroom/asparagus mix. Set aside. Cut or split a tiny sourdough loaf into 1-inch bits. (my loaf was a little too small, therefore that I used 4 challah rolls too) Grease a 9x13 inch baking dish and generate a base coating of bread at the dish. Spread 1/2 cup of fontina cheese on bread, at a coating, and disperse half green onions on the cheese. Lay-down a different layer of these vegetables and bread and a 1/2 cup of fontina cheese.

Whisk together eggs, salt, milk, dry mustard, and pepper into a bowl, and then pour the egg mixture on the vegetables and bread. Cover the dish, and then simmer for 3 hours. Preheat oven to 375 degrees. Remove the casserole from the fridge and let stand for half an hour. Spread all the parmesan cheese at a coating within the layers. Bake in the preheated oven until a knife inserted near the border comes out clean, 40 to 45 minutes. Let stand 5 to 10 minutes before cutting into squares.

Nutrition:

Calories: 349 Cal Fat: 18 g Fiber: 2 g Carbs: 25 g Protein: 22 g

11. Avocado Egg Toast

Preparation time: 0

Cooking time: 15 mins

Servings: 1

Ingredients:

¼ avocado

¼ tsp ground pepper 1/8 tsp garlic powder

One slice toasted whole-wheat bread one large boiled egg

1 tbsp sliced scallion

Directions:

Take a small bowl. Combine avocado, garlic, pepper in it gently. Top the toast with avocado mixture. Cut into half the egg. Place the egg on the top of the toast. If you want to garnish the toast with the scallion.

Nutrition: Calories: 298 Cal Fat: 24 g Fiber: 5 g Carbs: 18 g Protein: 19 g

12. Roll-Up Omelet with Spinach

Preparation time: 0

Cooking time: 40 mins

Servings: 1

Ingredients:

1 tsp canola oil one egg

1 cup baby spinach 1 tbsp olive tapenade

1 tbsp crumbled goat cheese

Directions:

Drizzle canola oil into a non-stick pan. Then, wipe with a paper towel. Heat the pan over medium heat. Beat egg and swirl into the frying pan. Cook 2 minutes. Then, flip the egg and cook 1 minute.

Carefully place the egg on a plate. In the same pan, sauté 1 cup of spinach about 1 minute, until wilted. Top the egg with olive tapenade and goat cheese. Then place wilted spinach on the ingredients. Roll up the egg and cut in half.

Nutrition:

Calories: 328 Cal

Fat: 12 g

Fiber: 5 g

Carbs: 31 g

Protein: 24 g

13. Avocado Chicken Roll

Preparation time: 0

Cooking time: 15 mins

Servings: 1

Ingredients:

0.22 lb fried chicken breast 1 tbsp mayonnaise

½ medium avocado,

0.16 lb salt and pepper

Directions:

Cut the chicken into long thin strips. Cut avocado into medium slices, put them in a plate, mix with mayonnaise and salt and pepper to taste. Put the avocado mixture on the meat strips. Roll strips.

Nutrition:

Calories: 246 Cal

Fat: 5 g

Fiber: 0 g

Carbs: 39 g

Protein: 8 g

14. Marinara Poached Egg

Preparation time: 0

Cooking time: 15 mins

Servings: 1

Ingredients:

2 tsp olive oil

¼ small yellow onion

A pinch of red pepper flakes

½ cup marinara sauce one egg

One small whole-wheat pita pocket

Directions:

Heat the olive oil in a small sauté pan over medium heat. Sauté the onion in the pan until brown, approximately 5 minutes. Add red pepper flakes and marinara sauce. Cook about 1 minute.

Gently break the egg into the pan. Cover the pan and simmer about 5 to 7 minutes until egg white is firm. Serve the dish with pita pocket. You can toast it and tear it into wedges.

Nutrition:

Calories: 148 Cal

Fat: 10 g

Fiber: 0 g

Carbs: 3 g

Protein: 13 g

15. Pita Pocket Sandwich

Preparation time: 0

Cooking time: 25 mins

Servings: 1

Ingredients:

One egg

One egg whites

½ tbsp milk

½ whole-wheat pita pocket, cut in half

½ cup baby spinach

Two grape tomatoes, sliced in half lengthwise

one green onions, diced

1/8 cup crumbles of Feta cheese 1 tsp olive oil

Directions:

Preheat oven to 340 °F. Whisk the eggs and egg whites with milk, tomatoes, and spinach in a medium mixing bowl. Add green onion, salt, and pepper to taste. Pour the mixture in a non-stick skillet. Cook the eggs for 15-18 minutes over medium-high heat. Sprinkle the top with feta cheese. Place in the oven for 1 minute. Brush each pita half with olive oil (both sides). Warm on the foil for 2 minutes. After baking, cut the omelette and place it on the pita.

Nutrition: Calories: 150 Cal Fat: 1 g

Fiber: 0 g Carbs: 12 g Protein: 8 g

16. Sesame Edamame

Preparation time: 0

Cooking time: 10 mins

Servings: 1

Ingredients:

1/2 tbsp water

3/4 cup edamame pods

1/3 tbsp light brown sugar

1/6 tbsp dark sesame oil

1/6 tbsp rice vinegar kosher

Salt to taste

Freshly ground black

Pepper to taste

1/4 tsp sesame seeds, toasted

Directions:

Boil water in a large frying pan over medium-high heat Add edamame to water. Cook 2 minutes.

Add sugar, vinegar, oil, salt, and pepper to edamame. Cook for 3- 5 minutes. Sprinkle with sesame seeds before serving.

Nutrition:

Calories: 100 Cal

Fat: 3 g

Fiber: 4 g

Carbs: 9 g

Protein: 8 g

17. Breakfast Roasted Veggie Frittata

Preparation time: 0

Cooking time: 1h 30 mins

Servings: 1

Ingredients:

1/2 medium bell peppers 1/2 garlic clove

1/3 large zucchini 1/6 medium onion 1/6 tbsp olive oil

1 tbsp cup fresh parsley, chopped 1 ½ egg

One egg whites salt to taste

Cayenne pepper to taste

2 tbsp finely shredded Parmesan Nonstick cooking spray

Directions:

Preheat oven to 400 °F. Place the first oven rack in the lowest position. The second track must be in the central location in the oven. Line two baking pans with foil. Spray the foil with cooking spray.

Place bell pepper and garlic on one pan. Place zucchini and onion on the other baking pan. Brush the products with olive oil. Place zucchini and onion on the centre rack and bake 15 minutes. Remove onion and zucchini. Place bell pepper and garlic on the lower rack—roast for 10 minutes.

Peel the bell pepper and garlic. Cut pepper into quarters. Cut the zucchini into three 1/2-

inch strips. Cut the onion into ½-inch slices. Chop the parsley. Shred the Parmesan. Place the vegetables and garlic in a bowl. Add parsley and ½ tsp of salt. Lower the heat in the oven to the 400 °F. Coat a 9-x-1.5-inch round cake pan (or smaller) with cooking spray. In a medium bowl, whisk eggs and egg whites. Add remaining salt and cayenne pepper. Add egg mixture to the vegetable mixture. Stir in Parmesan. Place the ingredients into the cake pan. Bake the mixture for 50 minutes. Let the frittata stand 15-30 min before serving.

Nutrition:

Calories: 139 Cal

Fat: 3 g

Fiber: 4 g

Carbs: 9 g

Protein: 8 g

Chapter 8:

Light Bites

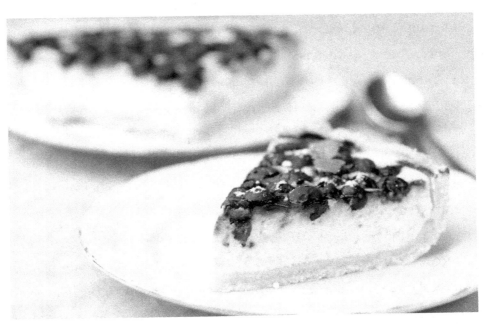

18. No-Bake Blueberry Cheesecake Bars

Preparation time: **15 minutes** (not including crust)

Cooking time: 7 minutes

Servings: 16

Ingredients:

2 (8-oz.) softened packages of Cream Cheese

1 Easy Shortbread Crust

¼ cup heavy whipping cream kept at room temp

½ cup of powdered Erythritol-based Sweetener

1 tsp grated Lemon Zest

Topping Ingredients: ¼ cup of Water

1 cup of Blueberries

1 tbsp fresh Lemon juice

¼ cup of powdered Erythritol-based Sweetener

¼ tsp Xanthan gum for garnish (optional)

Directions:

Preparing the Bars:

Firmly press the crust mixture of the shortbread into the bottom of a baking pan. Place the crust in the refrigerator. Melt the chocolate in a bowl that you've set over a pan that placed on the water that just began simmering. Take the bowl out of the pan and allow it to cool for about 10 minutes.

With an electric mixer, beat the sweetener and the butter for 2 minutes until it is well incorporated and fluffy. Carefully add the melted chocolate while the mixer is running and continue beating until smooth. Add the salt, espresso powder, and vanilla extract. Add in the eggs one after the other and continue beating for 5 minutes. Carefully pour the filling ingredients on the top of the chilled crust and make sure to smoothen the top. Refrigerate for 2 hours. Garnishing the Bars: Carefully spread the whipped cream and chocolate on top.

Nutrition: Fat: 23.7g Carbs: 4.6g Protein: 4.6g Fiber: 2.2g Calories: 255

19. Chocolate-Covered Cheesecake Bites

Preparation time: 20 minutes

Cooking time: 5 minutes

Servings: 12

Ingredients:

1 (8 oz.) package of softened Cream Cheese

½ stick (¼ cup) unsalted softened Butter

½ cup of powdered Erythritol-based Sweetener

½ tsp. of vanilla extract

4 oz. of sugarless chopped Dark Chocolate

1½ tbsp. of Coconut oil or ¾ oz. of Cacao Butter

Directions

Line a baking sheet with parchment or wax paper. Beat the butter and cream cheese with an electric mixer in a large bowl until it is thoroughly mixed. Beat in the vanilla extract and sweetener until smooth. Form the mixture into 1-inch balls and position on the coated baking sheet. Place them in the fridge for 3-4 hours until it becomes firm. Melt the cacao butter and chocolate together over water that just began simmering over a heatproof bowl. Stir until mixture becomes smooth. Remove from heat. Dunk each ball into melted chocolate. Coat thoroughly and remove using a fork. Firmly tap the fork on the sides of the bowl to eliminate extra chocolate. Position the ball on the baking sheet and let it set. Do the same for the rest of the cheesecake balls. Decoratively sprinkle the rest of the chocolate over the lined balls.

Nutrition:

Fat: 13.5g

Carbs: 5.2g

Protein: 1.7g

Fiber: 2.2g

Calories: 148

20. Delicious Italian Cake

Preparation Time: 10 minutes

Cooking Time: 55 minutes

Servings: 12

Ingredients:

Five eggs

2½ cups almond flour

1 tsp baking powder

1 cup unsweetened coconut flakes

2 tsp vanilla extract

2 cups Swerve confectioners' sugar

1 cup butter

1 tsp baking soda

1 cup sour cream

For frosting:

1 cup unsweetened coconut flakes

½ cup walnuts, chopped

2 Tbsp unsweetened almond milk

2 cups Swerve confectioners' sugar

1 tsp vanilla extract

½ cup butter

8 oz cream cheese

Directions:

Pour one cup of water into the Instant Pot and place a trivet in the pot. Spray a 7-inch cake pan with cooking spray and set aside. In a small bowl, mix sour cream and baking soda and set aside.

In a large bowl, whisk together 1 cup butter and the sweetener until fluffy. Mix the eggs, almond flour, baking powder, 1 cup coconut flakes, 2 tsp vanilla, and the sour cream mixture. Pour batter in the prepared cake pan—cover pan with aluminum foil. Place the cake pan on top of the trivet in the Instant Pot. Seal the pot with a lid and cook on manual mode for 35 minutes. When finished, allow pressure to release naturally for 20 minutes, and then release using the quick release method. Open the lid. Remove cake from the pot and let it cool completely. For the frosting: In a mixing bowl, beat together ½ cup butter, Swerve, cream cheese, and vanilla until fluffy. Add almond milk, walnuts, and coconut flakes and stir well. Spread the frosting on top of the cake. Slice and serve.

Nutrition:

Calories 591 Fat 57.6 g

Carbohydrates 11.3 g   Protein 11.9 g

21. Tiramisu Sheet Cake

Preparation time: 25 minutes

Cooking time: 22 minutes

Servings: 20

Ingredients:

¾ cup granulated Erythritol-based Sweetener

0.44 lb (2 cups) of blanched Almond flour

⅓ cup of unflavored Whey Protein powder

0.08 lb (⅓ cup) of Coconut flour

1 tbsp. of baking Powder

½ tsp. of salt

One stick (½ cup) of unsalted and melted butter

¾ cup of unsweetened Almond Milk

One tsp. of Vanilla extract

Three large eggs

One tbs. of dark Rum (optional)

¼ cup of cooled strong brewed coffee or espresso

Mascarpone Frosting Ingredients:

4 oz. (½ cup) of softened Cream Cheese

8 oz. of softened Mascarpone Cheese

One tsp. of Vanilla extract

A ½-⅔ cup of heavy Whipping cream kept at room temp

½ cup of powdered Erythritol-based Sweetener

Ingredients for Garnishing:

1-oz. of sugarless dark Chocolate

1 tbsp. of Cocoa powder

Directions:

In a blender or food processor, grind the macadamia nuts to a beautiful texture.

Add all the cinnamon roll ingredients except for caramel sauce, and then put in the refrigerator to chill for an hour.

Heat the oven to 350° F. Line a baking tray with parchment paper.

Roll out the dough and make a large rectangle shape on a parchment-lined surface.

Spread the Keto Caramel Sauce over the batter.

Carefully roll the dough into a log shape and seal the edge.

Place a sharp knife in warm water and cut the log into about 10-12 rolls.

Position rolls on coated tray and place in the oven for 25 to 30 minutes, making sure that you check after 20 minutes to check if it cooked through.

While the cinnamon rolls are baking in the oven, make the glaze. Combine all ingredients in a blender or mixing bowl.

Take keto cinnamon rolls out of the oven. Let it cool before you glaze. You can serve warm with glaze garnished on the top.

Nutrition:

Calories: 477 Fat: 45.6g Carbs: 17.1g
Fiber: 7.1g Protein: 5.6g

22. Cinnamon Crumb Cake Keto Donuts

Preparation time: 10 minutes
Cooking time: 15 minutes
Servings: 1
Ingredients:

½ cup of Coconut flour
¼ cup of Almond flour
1 tbsp of Flaxseed meal
1 tsp of baking powder
¼ tsp salt
1 tsp of Cinnamon
¼ tsp of Nutmeg
2/3 cup of Erythritol Sweetener (e.g. Swerve)
Six large eggs
½ cup of butter, melted
1 tsp of vanilla
½ cup of Almond flour
¼ cup of diced pecans (optional)
One pinch of salt
2 tbsp of softened butter

Directions:

Heat the oven to 350° F.

Use a non-stick spray to spray a doughnut pan.

Preparing the doughnuts:

Whisk the coconut flour, almond flour, flax meal, sweetener, baking powder, salt, nutmeg, and Cinnamon together inside a medium bowl. Set aside.

Whisk the eggs, vanilla, and melted butter until it appears. Add all the dry ingredients into wet ingredients and mix.

Spoon the batter into the doughnut space and fill it ¾ of the way full.

Preparing the crumb topping:

Stir together the sweetener, almond meal, and salt inside a small bowl. Add the butter and mix. Thoroughly mix until all of the flour is well combined, and the mixture moistened.

Topping the doughnuts:

Garnish the topping on the doughnuts, with fingers to break up the mixture until it is well mixed.

Place in the oven for 12-15 minutes or until the sides appear light brown.

Nutrition:

Calories: 138g Fat: 12g Carbs: 3g

Fiber: 2g Protein: 4g

23. Keto Espresso Chocolate Cheesecake Bars

Preparation time: 10 minutes

Cooking time: 35 minutes

Servings: 16

Ingredients:

7 tbsp. of melted Butter

2 cups of ultrafine, blanched Almond flour

3 tbsp. of Cocoa powder

1/3 cup granulated Erythritol sweetener

Cheesecake Ingredients:

16 oz. of full fat Cream Cheese

Two large eggs

½ cup of granulated Erythritol sweetener

2 tbsp. of instant Espresso powder

One tsp. of Vanilla extract

Extra cocoa powder for dusting over the top.

Directions:

Preparation o f the Chocolate Crust:

Heat the oven to 350° F.

Combine the almond flour, melted butter, cocoa powder, and sweetener in a medium-sized bowl.

Transfer the crust dough to a 9 x 9" pan coated with foil or parchment paper.

Firmly press the crust to the bottom of the pan.

Place the crust in the oven and bake for about 8 minutes.

Take out of the oven and set aside to cool.

Preparing the cheesecake filling:

Place the eggs, cream cheese, espresso powder, vanilla extract, and sweetener inside a blender and blend the mixture until smooth.

Pour over the crust and evenly spread out in the pan.

Bake for 25 minutes. Take out of the oven and allow it to cool. Dust it with the cocoa powder

Place in the refrigerator to chill. Afterwards, cut into four rows of squares to serve.

Nutrition:

Calories: 232 Fat: 21g

Carbs: 5g Fiber: 1.5g

Protein: 6g

24. Mini No-Bake Lemon Cheesecakes

Preparation time: 20 minutes

Cooking time: 0

Servings: 6

Ingredients:

½ cup of blanched almond flour

2 tbsp. of powdered Erythritol-based Sweetener

⅛ tsp. of salt

2 tbsp. unsalted and melted butter

Filling:

One tbs. plus ¼ cup powdered Erythritol-based Sweetener

¾ cup (6 oz.) of softened Cream Cheese

¼ cup of heavy whipping cream kept at room temp

½ tsp. of Lemon extract

Two tsp. of grated Lemon Zest

2 tbsp. of fresh Lemon juice

Directions:

Preparing the Crust Ingredients:

Line muffin pan with parchment paper or silicone.

Whisk the sweetener, almond flour. Add the melted butter and stir until mixture starts clumping together.

Place the crust in the muffin cups you've prepared and made sure to press into the bottoms firmly.

Preparing the Filling:

With an electric mixer, beat the cream cheese in a medium bowl. Add the sweetener until it is well combined.

Beat in the lemon extract, lemon juice, lemon zest, and the cream until smooth.

Share the filling mixture into the muffin cups you prepared and fill all of the containers to almost the top. Also, smoothen the top. To let go of air bubbles firmly tap the pan on a counter.

For 2 hours, place the pan in the fridge so that the filling becomes firm. Carefully remove the silicone layers or the parchment paper liners. Serve when ready.

Nutrition:

Fat: 20.1g

Carbs: 3.9g

Protein: 4g

Fiber: 1.1g

Calories: 223

25. Baked Maple Apple

Preparation time: 10 minutes

Cooking time: 30 minutes

Servings: 2

Ingredients:

Two small apples

Two teaspoons reduced-calorie apricot spread (16 calories per 2teaspoons)

One teaspoon reduced-calorie maple-flavored syrup (60 calories per fluid ounce)

Directions:

Remove the core from each apple to 1/2 inch from the bottom. Remove a thin strip of peel from around the center of each apple (this helps keep skin from bursting). Fill each apple with one teaspoon apricot spread and 1/2 teaspoon maple syrup. Place each apple upright in individual baking dish; cover dishes with foil and bake at 400°F until apples are tender, 25 to 30 minutes.

Nutrition:

75 calories.

0.2 g protein.

1 g fat.

19 g carbohydrate.

0.3 mg sodium.

0 mg cholesterol

26. Apple-Raisin Cake

This cake may be frozen for future use; to make serving easier, slice cake into individual portions, then wrap each portion in plastic freezer wrap and freeze. When ready to use, thaw the number of portions needed at room temperature.

Preparation time: 10 minutes

Cooking time: 50 minutes

Servings: 12

Ingredients:

One teaspoon baking soda

1/2 cups applesauce (no sugar added)

Two small Golden Delicious apples, cored, pared, and shredded

1 cup less 2 tablespoons raisins

2/4 cups self-rising flour

1 teaspoon ground cinnamon

1/2 teaspoon ground cloves 1/3 cup plus 2 teaspoons unsalted margarine

1/4 cup granulated sugar

Directions:

Spray an 8 x 8 x 2-inch baking pan with nonstick cooking spray and set aside. Into a medium bowl sift together flour, cinnamon, and cloves; set aside.

Preheat oven to 350°F. In a medium mixing bowl, using an electric mixer, cream margarine, add sugar and stir to combine. Stir baking soda into applesauce, then add to margarine mixture and stir to combine; add sifted ingredients and, using an electric mixer on medium speed, beat until thoroughly combined. Fold in apples and raisins; pour batter into the sprayed pan and bake for 45 to 50 minutes (until cake is browned and a cake tester or toothpick, inserted in center, comes out dry). Remove cake from pan and cool on wire rack.

Nutrition:

151 calories.

2 g protein.

4 g fat.

28 g carbohydrate.

96 mg sodium.

0 mg cholesterol

27. Cinnamon-Apricot Bananas

Preparation time: 10 minutes

Cooking time: 20 minutes

Servings: 2

Ingredients:

4 graham crackers 2x2-inch 1 medium banana, peeled and cut in squares), made into crumbs half lengthwise

2 teaspoons shredded coconut

1/4 teaspoon ground cinnamon

1 tablespoon plus 1 teaspoon reduced-calorie apricot spread (16 calories per 2 teaspoons)

Directions:

In small skillet combine crumbs, coconut, and cinnamon and toast lightly, being careful not to burn; transfer to a sheet of wax paper or a paper plate and set aside.

In the same skillet heat apricot spread until melted; remove from heat. Roll each banana half in a spread, then quickly roll in crumb mixture, pressing crumbs so that they adhere to the banana; place coated halves on a plate, cover lightly, and refrigerate until chilled.

Variation: Coconut-Strawberry Bananas — Omit cinnamon and substitute reduced-calorie strawberry spread (16 calories per 2 teaspoons) for the apricot spread.

Nutrition:

130 calories.

2 g protein.

2 g fat.

29 g carbohydrate.

95 mg sodium.

0 mg cholesterol

28. Meringue Crepes with Blueberry Custard Filling

Preparation time: 10 minutes

Cooking time: 20 minutes

Servings: 4

Ingredients:

2 cups blueberries (reserve 8 berries for garnish)

8 crepes

1 cup evaporated skimmed milk

2 large eggs, separated

1 tablespoon plus 1 teaspoon

granulated sugar, divided

2 teaspoons each cornstarch

lemon juice

Directions:

In 1-quart saucepan, combine milk, egg yolks, and one tablespoon sugar; cook over low heat, continually stirring, until slightly thickened and bubbles form around sides of the mixture. In a cup or small bowl dissolve cornstarch in lemon juice; gradually stir into milk mixture and cook, constantly stirring, until thick. Remove from heat and fold in blueberries; let cool.

Spoon Vs. of custard onto the center of each crepe and fold sides over filling to enclose; arrange crepes, seam-side down, in an 8 x 8 x 2-inch baking pan. In a small bowl, using an electric mixer on high speed, beat egg whites until soft peaks form; add remaining teaspoon sugar, and continue beating until stiff peaks form.

Fill the pastry bag with egg whites and pipe an equal amount over each crepe (if pastry bag is not available, spoon egg whites over crepes); top each with a reserved blueberry and broil until meringue is lightly browned, 10 to 15 seconds. Serve immediately.

Nutrition:

300 calories.

16 g protein.

6 g fat.

45 g carbohydrate.

180 mg sodium.

278 mg cholesterol

29. Meatless Borscht

Preparation time: 10 minutes

Cooking time: 25 minutes

Servings: 2

Ingredients:

1 teaspoon margarine

1 cup shredded green cabbage

1/4 cup chopped onion

1/4 cup sliced carrot

1 cup coarsely shredded pared

2 tablespoons tomato paste beets

1 tablespoon lemon juice

2 cups of water

1/2 teaspoon granulated sugar

2 packets instant beef broth and 1 teaspoon pepper

seasoning mix

1/4 cup plain low-fat yogurt

1/2 bay leaf

Directions:

In 1 1/2-quart saucepan heat margarine until bubbly and hot; add onion and saute until softened, 1 to 2 minutes. Add beets and toss to combine; add water, broth mix, and bay leaf and bring to a boil. Cover pan and cook over medium heat for 10 minutes; stir in remaining ingredients except for yogurt, cover, and let simmer until vegetables are tender about 25 minutes. Remove and discard bay leaf. Pour borscht into 2 soup bowls and top each portion with 2 tablespoons yogurt.

Nutrition:

120 calories.

5 g protein.

3 g fat.

21 g carbohydrate.

982 mg sodium.

2 mg cholesterol

30. Sauteed Sweet 'n' Sour Beets

Preparation time: 5 minutes

Cooking time: 10 minutes

Servings: 2

Ingredients:

2 teaspoons margarine

1 tablespoon diced onion

1 cup drained canned small whole beets, cut into quarters

1 tablespoon each lemon juice and water

1 teaspoon each salt and pepper

Dash granulated sugar substitute

Directions:

In small nonstick skillet heat margarine over medium-high heat until bubbly and hot; add onion and saute until softened, 1 to 2 minutes. Reduce heat to low and add remaining ingredients; cover pan and cook, stirring once, for 5 minutes longer.

Nutrition:

70 calories.

1 g protein.

4 g fat.

9 g carbohydrate.

385 mg sodium.

0 mg cholesterol

31. Orange Beets

Preparation time: 5 minutes

Cooking time: 20 minutes

Servings: 2

Ingredients:

1 /2 teaspoons lemon juice

1 teaspoon cornstarch Dash salt

1 teaspoon orange marmalade

1 cup peeled and sliced cooked beets

2 teaspoons margarine

1 teaspoon firmly packed brown

sugar 1/4 cup orange juice (no sugar added)

Directions:

In a 1-quart saucepan (not aluminum or cast-iron), combine beets, margarine, and sugar; cook over low heat, continually stirring until margarine and sugar are melted.

In 1-cup measure or small bowl combine juices, cornstarch, and salt, stirring to dissolve cornstarch; pour over beet mixture and, constantly stirring, bring to a boil. Continue cooking and stirring until the mixture thickens.

Reduce heat, add marmalade, and stir until combined. Remove from heat and let cool slightly; cover and refrigerate for at least 1 hour. Reheat before serving.

Nutrition:

99 calories.

1 g protein.

4 g fat.

16 g carbohydrate.

146 mg sodium.

0 mg cholesterol

32. Cabbage 'n' Potato Soup

This soup freezes well; for easy portion control, freeze in pre-measured servings.

Preparation time: 10 minutes

Cooking time: 30 minutes

Servings: 4

Ingredients:

2 teaspoons vegetable oil

4 cups shredded green cabbage

1 cup sliced onions

1 garlic clove, minced

3 cups of water

6 ounces peeled potato, sliced

1 cup each sliced carrot and tomato puree

4 packets instant beef broth and seasoning mix

1 each bay leaf and whole clove

Directions:

In 2-quart saucepan heat oil, add cabbage, onions, and garlic and saute over medium heat, frequently stirring, until cabbage is soft, about 10 minutes. Reduce heat to low and add remaining ingredients; cook until vegetables are tender, about 30 minutes. Remove and discard bay leaf and clove before serving.

Nutrition:

119 calories.

4 g protein.

3 g fat.

22 g carbohydrate.

900 mg sodium,

0 mg cholesterol.

33. Eggplant Pesto

Preparation time: 10 minutes

Cooking time: 40 minutes

Servings: 2

Ingredients:

1 medium eggplant (about 1 pound), cut crosswise into thick rounds

Dash salt

2 tablespoons each chopped

Fresh basil and grated Parmesan cheese

1 tablespoon olive oil

1 small garlic clove, mashed

Dash freshly ground pepper

Directions:

On 10 X 15-inch nonstick baking sheet arrange eggplant slices in a single layer; sprinkle with salt and bake at 425°F. until easily pierced with a fork, about 30 minutes.

In a small bowl, combine remaining ingredients; spread an equal amount of mixture over each eggplant slice. Transfer slices to I1/2-quart casserole, return to oven, and bake until heated, about 10 minutes longer.

Nutrition:

144 calories. 5 g protein.

9 g fat. 14 g carbohydrate.

163 mg sodium. 4 mg cholesterol

34. Ratatouille

Preparation time: 10 minutes

Cooking time: 40 minutes

Servings: 4

Ingredients:

1 tablespoon plus 1 teaspoon olive oil

1 cup each sliced onion and red or green bell peppers

3 garlic cloves, chopped

4 cups cubed eggplant (1-inch cubes)

1/2 cups canned Italian tomatoes, chopped 1 cup sliced zucchini

3 tablespoons chopped fresh basil or 2 teaspoons dried

1 teaspoon salt

Dash freshly ground pepper

Directions:

In 12-inch skillet heat oil over medium heat; add onions, bell peppers, and garlic and saute until vegetables are tender-crisp. Add remaining ingredients and stir to combine. Reduce heat, cover, and let simmer until vegetables are tender, 20 to 25 minutes.

Variations:

Use Ratatouille as an omelet filling.

Place Ratatouille in 10 x 6 x 2-inch baking dish; top with 4 ounces shredded hard cheese and bake at 350°F. until cheese is melted.

Nutrition:

237 calories. 11 g protein.

15 g fat.

18 g carbohydrate.

842 mg sodium.

30 mg cholesterol

35. Chilled Eggplant Relish

Preparation time: 10 minutes

Cooking time: 20 minutes

Servings: 4

Ingredients:

3 cups cubed eggplant

1 teaspoon salt

1 tablespoon plus

1 teaspoon olive oil

1 cup thinly sliced onions

2 garlic cloves, minced

1 cup each diced celery and chopped tomatoes

2 teaspoons wine vinegar

1 teaspoon granulated sugar

8 black olives, pitted and cut into halves

1 tablespoon drained capers

Directions:

On paper towels arrange eggplant in a single layer; sprinkle with salt and let stand for at least 1 hour. Pat dry and set aside.

In 9- or 10-inch skillet heat oil over medium heat; add onions and garlic and saute until onions are translucent, 3 to 5 minutes. Add eggplant and cook, occasionally stirring, until eggplant begins to soften, about 5 minutes; stir in celery and tomatoes, cover pan, and let simmer until celery is tender about 15 minutes.

Stir in vinegar and sugar and cook, uncovered, for 5 minutes longer. Remove from heat and add olives and capers, tossing to combine; transfer to a glass, plastic, or stainless-steel container, cover, and refrigerate until chilled.

Nutrition:

113 calories.

3 g protein.

7 g fat.

13 g carbohydrate.

429 mg sodium.

0 mg cholesterol

36. Endive-Tomato Salad with Sesame Dressing

Preparation time: 40 minutes

Cooking time: 0

Servings: 2

Ingredients:

Salad:

5 medium Belgian endives (about 3 ounces each)

2 cup chopped watercress leaves

o6 cherry tomatoes, cut into quarters

Dressing:

1 teaspoon each sesame seed, toasted, lemon juice, rice vinegar, and water

2 garlic cloves, mashed

Dash salt

Directions:

To Prepare Salad: Separate each endive into individual leaves. Line a clear 1-quart salad bowl with endive leaves with tips facing rim of bowl-like flower petals. Fill center of the bowl with chopped watercress; top watercress with cherry tomato quarters, arranged in a circular pattern. Refrigerate for at least 30 minutes.

To Prepare Dressing: Using a mortar and pestle, mash sesame seed. In a small bowl or cup, combine mashed grain with lemon juice, vinegar, water, garlic, and salt; mix well. Refrigerate for at least 30 minutes.

To Serve: Stir dressing and pour over salad.

Nutrition:

50 calories. 3 g protein.

1 g fat. 9 g carbohydrate. 86 mg sodium.

0 mg cholesterol

Chapter 9:

Main Meals

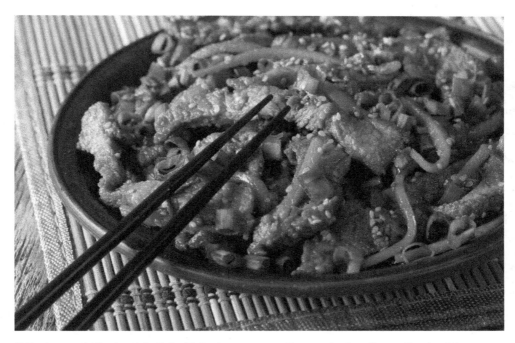

37. Miso Marinated Cod with Stir-Fried Greens and Sesame

Preparation time: 20 minutes

Cooking time: 0

Servings: 1

Ingredients:

Skinless cod fillet - 1 x 7-ounce

Mirin - 1 tablespoon

Miso - 3 ½ teaspoon

Kale - ¾ cup (roughly chopped)

Extra virgin olive oil - 1 tablespoon

Red onion - 1/8 cup (sliced)

Celery - 3/8 cup (sliced)

Buckwheat - ¼ cup

Bird's eye chili – 1 (finely chopped)

Garlic clove - 1 (finely chopped)

Finely chopped fresh ginger - 1 teaspoon

Sesame seeds - 1 teaspoon

Green beans - 3/8 cup

Parsley - 2 tablespoon (roughly chopped)

Tamari - 1 tablespoon

Ground turmeric - 1 teaspoon

Directions:

Add one teaspoon of oil, the mirin and miso into a bowl and mix together. Rub the mixture all over the cod and leave it for 30 minutes to marinate. Heat your oven to 220°C or 425°F. bake the cod for approx. ten minutes.

Add the remaining oil into a large frypan or wok over medium heat. Once hot, add the onions and stir-fry for 3 minutes, then add the garlic, celery, green beans, ginger, chili, and kale. Stir and fry until the kale is well cooked and tender. Add a little water to the pan if needed to aid the cooking process.

Cook the buckwheat following the instruction on the packet, add the turmeric three minutes to the end.

Add the sesame seeds, tamari, and parsley to the stir fry. Serve with the fish and the greens.

Nutrition:

Calories: 185 Cal Fat: 2 g

Fiber: 1 g Carbs: 17 g Protein: 25 g

38. Kale and Turmeric Chicken Salad and Honey Lime Dressing

Preparation time: 20 mins

Cooking Time: 10 mins

Servings: 2

Ingredients

For the Chicken

Chicken thighs – 9 oz./ 300 g (diced)

Coconut oil – 1 tablespoon, or ghee – 1 teaspoon

Turmeric powder – 1 teaspoon

Medium brown onion – ½ (diced)

Large garlic clove – 1 (finely chopped)

Juice of a half lime

Lime zest – 1 teaspoon

Pepper and salt, to taste – ½ teaspoon

For the Salad

A handful of fresh parsley leaves – chopped

A handful of fresh coriander leaves – chopped

Kale – 3 large leaves (stems removed, and leaves chopped)

Pumpkin seeds – 2 tablespoons

Broccoli florets – 2 cups, or broccolini stalks – 6

Avocado – ½ (sliced)

For the Dressing

Raw honey – 1 teaspoon

Lime juice – 3 tablespoons

Pepper and sea salt, to taste – ½ teaspoon

Dijon mustard or wholegrain – ½ teaspoon

Small garlic clove – 1 (grated or finely diced)

Extra-virgin olive oil – 3 tablespoons

Directions:

Get your chicken ready. Heat your coconut oil in a small frypan over medium-high heat. Add the chopped onion and sauté until golden, this will take about five minutes. Add the garlic and the diced chicken, stir for another two to three minutes to break it apart.

Add the lime juice and zest, turmeric powder, pepper, and salt and cook for another four minutes, stirring occasionally. Set aside once the time is up.

While cooking the chicken, add water to a small saucepan and allow to boil. Add the broccolini once the water is boiled and cook for approx. two minutes. Rinse the vegetable under cold water and cut into 3 or 4 pieces each.

Add the pumpkin seeds to a dry frypan and toast over medium heat for approx. two minutes, while occasionally stirring to prevent the seeds from getting burnt. Season with a little salt. Set aside. You may also use the pumpkin seeds raw if you want.

Add the chopped kale into your salad bowl and pour over your dressing. Use your fingers to massage and toss the kale with the dressing to soften the kale.

Now add the sliced avocado, pumpkin seeds, broccolini, cooked chicken, fresh parsley, and coriander leaves. Toss together. Serve.

Note: You may use chopped fish, prawn, or beef mince in place of the chicken.

Nutrition:

Calories: 230 Cal Fat: 13 g Fiber: 3 g

Carbs: 18 g Protein: 11 g

39. Sirt Chili Con Carne

Preparation time: 45 mins

Cooking Time: 45 mins

Servings: 4

Ingredients:

Buckwheat – 5.6oz

Lean minced beef (5% fat) – 14 oz

Beef stock – 0.08 gallon

Red onion - 1 (finely chopped)

Garlic cloves - 3 (finely chopped)

Extra virgin olive oil - 1 tablespoon

Bird's eye chilies - 2 (finely chopped)

Ground turmeric - 1 tablespoon

Ground cumin - 1 tablespoon

Red wine - 5 oz

Tomato purée - 1 tablespoon

Red pepper – 1 (cored, seeds removed and cut into bite-sized pieces)

Chopped tomatoes - 2 x 14.1 oz tins

Cocoa powder - 1 tablespoon

Tinned kidney beans – 1 cup

Parsley – 1 teaspoon (chopped)

Coriander - 1 teaspoon (chopped)

Directions:

Place a casserole over medium heat. Once the oil gets hot, add the oil, then add the onion, chili, and garlic—Fry for about 3 minutes.

Increase the heat to high, then add the minced beef to the pan and allow it to brown. Now add the red wine and allow to bubble to reduce it by half.

Add the tomatoes, cocoa, red pepper, tomato purée and stock to the casserole and leave to simmer for approx. one hour.

Add a little water if the consistency is too thick and sticky.

Stir in the chopped herbs just before you serve.

Cook the buckwheat following the instruction on the packet and serve together with the chili.

Nutrition: Calories: 320 Cal Fat: 21 g Fiber: 4 g Carbs: 8 g Protein: 24 g

40. Chickpea Turmeric Stew with Coconut Bacon

Preparation time: 30 mins

Cooking Time: 30 mins

Servings: 2

Ingredients:

For the Chickpea Turmeric Stew:

Minced fresh ginger – 1 tablespoon

Extra virgin olive oil – 3 tablespoons

Medium potato – 1 (cubed)

Minced fresh turmeric root – 2 tablespoons

Garlic – 3 cloves (minced)

Shallot – 1 (minced)

Mild curry powder – ½ tablespoon

Serrano peppers – 1 or 2 (finely chopped)

Pineapple juice – ½ cup

Coconut milk – 1 ½ cups

Lime juice – 2 tablespoons

Chickpeas – 1 ½ cups

Soy sauce – 2 teaspoons

Small sweet potato – 1 (cubed)

Salt, to taste

Chopped green onion or cilantro, for serving

Rice for serving.

For the Coconut Bacon

Honey – ½ tablespoon

Pineapple juice – ½ tablespoon

Soy sauce – 1 tablespoon

Unsweetened coconut flakes – 1 ½ cups

Liquid smoke – ¼ teaspoon

Thai red curry paste – 2 teaspoons

Directions:

For the Coconut bacon

Heat your oven to 275 degrees F. Place parchment paper on a baking sheet, then pour the flaked coconut into the baking sheet.

Add the rest of the ingredients for the coconut bacon into a small bowl and whisk together, ensure that all the ingredients are well mixed.

Drizzle the mixture over the coconut and use your fingers to coat the coconut. Spread out the coconuts in an even layer, then place in the oven to bake for approx. twenty minutes, or until the coconut is evenly browned and the liquid is absorbed. Stir every 5 minutes.

Keep aside to cool before using. You can also store it in an airtight container at room temperature for up to one week.

For the Chickpea Turmeric Stew:

Place a saucepan over medium heat and drizzle small olive oil into the pan. Once the oil begins to shimmer, add the shallot, and sprinkle some salt. Cook for about two minutes, until soft. Then add the turmeric, pepper, ginger, a sprinkle of salt and the garlic.

Stir and allow to cook for another 3 minutes until the shallot is soft. Now add the curry powder and cook for another one minute, stirring occasionally.

Stir in the pineapple juice, cubed potatoes, soy sauce and coconut milk, then sprinkle another pinch of salt.

Allow the mixture to boil gently, then reduce the heat to a simmer and cover with a lid.

Cook for another 20 minutes or until the potatoes are well cooked.

You may use the back of your spoon to mash some of the potatoes if you want your soup to be slightly thick. Stir in the lime juice and the cooked chickpeas and allow to simmer for another five minutes, partially cover.

Adjust the seasoning if needed.

Garnish with coconut bacon and cilantro.

Nutrition:

Calories: 303 Cal

Fat: 20 g

Fiber: 6 g

Carbs: 27 g

Protein: 6 g

41. Chinese-Style Pork with Pak Choi

Preparation time: 0 mins

Cooking Time: 30 mins

Servings: 4

Ingredients:

Firm tofu – 14 ounces (cut into large cubes)

Water - 1 tablespoon

Corn flour - 1 tablespoon

Chicken stock – 4.4 fl oz

Tomato purée - 1 tablespoon

Rice wine - 1 tablespoon

Soy sauce - 1 tablespoon

Brown sugar - 1 teaspoon

Fresh ginger - 1 thumb (peeled and grated)

Garlic - 1 clove (peeled and crushed)

Shiitake mushrooms - 3.5 ounces (sliced)

Choi sum or Pak choy – 7 ounces (cut into thin slices)

Beansprouts – 3.5 ounces

Rapeseed oil - 1 tablespoon

Parsley – a large handful (chopped)

Shallot – 1 (peeled and sliced)

Pork mince (10% fat) – 7 ounces

Directions:

Place the tofu on a kitchen paper, then cover the tofu with another kitchen paper, and set aside.

Add the water and corn flour in a bowl and mix together, removing all lumps. Then add the rice wine, soy sauce, tomato puree, chicken stock, and brown sugar. Stir. Lastly, add the crushed ginger and garlic and stir together.

In a large frypan or wok, add the oil and heat to a high temperature. Add the shiitake mushrooms to the pan and stir-fry for about 3 minutes until glossy and cooked. Use a slotted spoon to remove the mushrooms and keep aside.

Add the Pak choy and shallots to the frypan and stir-fry for two minutes, then add the mince. Cook until the mince is well done, then add the sauce. Reduce the heat a little and allow the sauce to bubble round the meat for about two minutes. Add the tofu, shiitake mushrooms and beansprout to the pan, stir and warm through. Put off the heat, then add the parsley. Stir before serving.

Nutrition:

Calories: 331 Cal

Fat: 11 g

Fiber: 0 g

Carbs: 28 g

Protein: 28 g

42. Tuscan Bean Stew

Preparation time: 0 mins

Cooking Time: 40 mins

Servings: 2 -3

Ingredients:

Chopped Italian tomatoes – 0.88 lb tin x 1

Buckwheat – 1.5 ounces

Extra virgin olive oil - 1 tablespoon

Vegetable stock - 6.7 ounces

Red onion - ¾ cup (finely chopped)

Carrot – ¼ cup (peeled and finely chopped)

Herbies de Provence - 1 teaspoon

Celery – 1 ounce (trimmed and finely chopped)

Garlic clove - 1 (finely chopped)

Tinned mixed beans – 1 cup

Bird's eye chili - ½ (finely chopped), optional

Tomato purée - 1 teaspoon

Roughly chopped parsley - 1 tablespoon

Kale – ½ cup (roughly chopped)

Directions:

Pour the oil into a medium saucepan over low-medium heat. Once hot, add the onion, celery, carrot, herbs, garlic, and chili and stir fry until the onion gets soft but not colored. Add the tomatoes, stock, and the tomato puree to the pan and bring to a boil. Add the beans and allow to simmer for thirty minutes.

Add the kale and cook for an additional 5 to 10 minutes, until tender. Now add the parsley. Cook the buckwheat following the instructions on the packet. Drain the water, then serve with the stew.

Nutrition:

Calories: 280 Cal

Fat: 9 g

Fiber: 23 g

Carbs: 36 g

Protein: 13 g

Chapter 10:

Smoothies

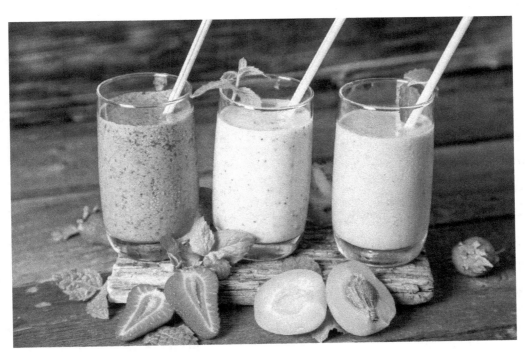

43. Apple and Cinnamon Smoothie

Preparation time: 5 mins

Cooking Time: 0 mins

Servings: 2

Ingredients:

2 apples, peeled, cored, sliced

4 tablespoons pecans

4 Medjool dates, pitted

½ teaspoon vanilla extract, unsweetened

2 cups almond milk, unsweetened

Extra:

1 ½ tablespoon ground cinnamon

Directions

Place all the ingredients in the order into a food processor or blender, and then pulse for 1 to 2 minutes until smooth.

Distribute smoothie between two glasses and then serve.

Meal Prep Instructions:

Divide smoothie between two jars or bottles, cover with a lid and then store the containers in the refrigerator for up to 3 days.

Nutrition:

Calories: 363 Cal Fat: 12 g

Fiber: 0 g Carbs: 36 g Protein: 60 g

44. Peanut Butter Cup Protein Shake

Preparation time: 5 mins

Cooking Time: 0 mins

Servings: 2

Ingredients:

1 banana, peeled

1 scoop of chocolate protein powder

1 tablespoon nutritional yeast

2 tablespoons peanut butter

½ cup almond milk, unsweetened

Extra:

½ teaspoon turmeric powder

Directions:

Place all the ingredients in the order into a food processor or blender, and then pulse for 1 to 2 minutes until smooth.

Distribute smoothie between two glasses and then serve.

Meal Prep Instructions:

Divide smoothie between two jars or bottles, cover with a lid, and then store the containers in the refrigerator for up to 3 days.

Nutrition:

Calories: 233 Cal Fat: 11.1 g

Fiber: 0 g Carbs: 18.6 g Protein: 14.6 g

45. Strawberry, Mango and Yogurt Smoothie

Preparation time: 5 mins

Cooking Time: 10 mins

Servings: 2

Ingredients:

1 mango, destoned, peeled, diced

4 ounces strawberries

1.3 ounces yogurt

2 cups almond milk, unsweetened

Directions

Place all the ingredients in the order into a food processor or blender, and then pulse for 1 to 2 minutes until smooth.

Distribute smoothie between two glasses and then serve.

Nutrition:

Calories: 166.5 Cal Fat: 3.7 g

Fiber: 3.8 g Carbs: 30.4 g Protein: 3.3 g

46. Berries Vanilla Protein Smoothie

Preparation time: 5 mins

Cooking Time: 0 mins

Servings: 2

Ingredients:

2 ounces blackberries

2 ounces strawberries

2 ounces raspberries

2 scoops of vanilla protein powder

1 ½ cup almond milk, unsweetened

Directions

Place all the ingredients in the order into a food processor or blender, and then pulse for 1 to 2 minutes until smooth.

Distribute smoothie between two glasses and then serve.

Meal Prep Instructions:

Divide smoothie between two jars or bottles, cover with a lid and then store the containers in the refrigerator for up to 3 days.

Nutrition

Calories: 151 Cal

Fat: 2.8 g Fiber: 4.4 g

Carbs: 10.9 g Protein: 20.3 g

47. Peanut Butter and Strawberry Smoothie

Preparation time: 5 mins

Cooking Time: 0 mins

Servings: 2

Ingredients:

2 ounces strawberry

2 bananas, peeled, sliced

2 tablespoons peanut butter

1 ½ cup almond milk, unsweetened

Directions

Place all the ingredients in the order into a food processor or blender, and then pulse for 1 to 2 minutes until smooth.

Distribute smoothie between two glasses and then serve.

Meal Prep Instructions:

Divide smoothie between two jars or bottles, cover with a lid and then store the containers in the refrigerator for up to 3 days.

Nutrition:

Calories: 238 Cal

Fat: 9.8 g

Fiber: 4.5 g

Carbs: 32.1 g

Protein: 5.3 g

48. Cherry and Vanilla Protein Shake

Preparation time: 5 mins

Cooking Time: 10 mins

Servings: 2

Ingredients:

4 ounces cherries, destemmed

1 scoop vanilla protein powder

1 ½ cup almond milk, unsweetened

Directions

Place all the ingredients in the order into a food processor or blender, and then pulse for 1 to 2 minutes until smooth.

Distribute shake between two glasses and then serve.

Meal Prep Instructions:

Divide shake between two jars or bottles, cover with a lid, and then store the containers in the refrigerator for up to 3 days.

Nutrition:

Calories: 193 Cal

Fat: 8 g

Fiber: 11 g

Carbs: 38 g

Protein: 5.2 g

49. Sirt Food Cocktail

Preparation time: 5 mins

Cooking Time: 0 mins

Servings: 1

Ingredients:

3oz kale

2oz strawberries

1 apple, cored

2 sticks of celery

1 tablespoon parsley

1 teaspoon of matcha powder

Squeeze lemon juice (optional) to taste

Directions:

Place the ingredients into a blender and add enough water to cover the ingredients and blitz to a smooth consistency.

Nutrition:

Calories: 101 Cal

Fat: 1 g

Fiber: 1 g

Carbs: 12 g

Protein: 10 g

50. Summer Berry Smoothie

Preparation time: 5 mins

Cooking Time: 0 mins

Servings: 1

Ingredients:

2oz blueberries

2oz strawberries

1oz blackcurrants

1oz red grapes

1 carrot, peeled

1 orange, peeled

Juice of 1 lime

Directions:

Place all of the ingredients into a blender and cover them with water. Blitz until smooth. You can also add some crushed ice and a mint leaf to garnish.

Nutrition:

Calories: 367 Cal

Fat: 7 g

Fiber: 5 g

Carbs: 0 g

Protein: 19 g

51. Mango, Celery & Ginger Smoothie

Preparation time: 5 mins

Cooking Time: 0 mins

Servings: 1

Ingredients:

1 stalk of celery

2oz kale

1 apple, cored

2oz mango, peeled, de-stoned and chopped

1 inch chunk of fresh ginger root, peeled and chopped

Directions:

Put all the ingredients into a blender with some water and blitz until smooth. Add ice to make your smoothie really refreshing.

Nutrition:

Calories: 105 Cal

Fat: 0.8 g

Fiber: 3.5 g

Carbs: 26.4 g

Protein: 2.5 g

52. Orange, Carrot & Kale Smoothie

Preparation time: 5 mins

Cooking Time: 0 mins

Servings: 1

Ingredients:

1 carrot, peeled

1 orange, peeled

1 stick of celery

1 apple, cored

2oz kale

½ teaspoon matcha powder

Directions:

Place all of the ingredients into a blender and add in enough water to cover them. Process until smooth, serve and enjoy.

Nutrition:

Calories: 156 Cal Fat: 1 g

Fiber: 7 g Carbs: 68 g

Protein: 5 g

53. Creamy Strawberry & Cherry Smoothie

Preparation time: 5 mins

Cooking Time: 0 mins

Servings: 1

Ingredients:

3½ oz strawberries

3oz frozen pitted cherries

1 tablespoon plain full-fat yogurt

6fl oz unsweetened soya milk

Directions:

Place all of the ingredients into a blender and process until smooth. Serve and enjoy.

Nutrition:

Calories: 132 Cal Fat: g Fiber: g

Carbs: g Protein: g

54. Pineapple & Cucumber Smoothie

Preparation time: 5 mins

Cooking Time: 0 mins

Servings: 1

Ingredients:

2oz cucumber

1 stalk of celery

2 slices of fresh pineapple

2 sprigs of parsley

½ teaspoon matcha powder

Squeeze of lemon juice

Serves 1

77 calories per serving

Directions:

Place all of the ingredients into blender with enough water to cover them and blitz until smooth.

Nutrition:

Calories: 77 Cal Fat: g Fiber: g

Carbs: g Protein: g

55. Avocado, Celery & Pineapple Smoothie

Preparation time: 5 mins

Cooking Time: 0 mins

Servings: 1

Ingredients:

2oz fresh pineapple, peeled and chopped

3 stalks of celery

1 avocado, peeled & de-stoned

1 teaspoon fresh parsley

½ teaspoon matcha powder

Juice of ½ lemon

Directions:

Place all of the ingredients into a blender and add enough water to cover them. Process until creamy and smooth.

Nutrition: Calories: 306 Cal Fat: 0 g Fiber: 15 g Carbs: 49 g Protein: 8 g

56. Mango & Rocket (Arugula) Smoothie

Preparation time: 5 mins

Cooking Time: 0 mins

Servings: 1

Ingredients:

1oz fresh rocket (arugula)

5oz fresh mango, peeled, de-stoned and chopped

1 avocado, de-stoned and peeled

½ teaspoon matcha powder

Juice of 1 lime

Directions:

Place all of the ingredients into a blender with enough water to cover them and process until smooth. Add a few ice cubes and enjoy.

Nutrition:

Calories: 369 Cal

Fat: 0 g

Fiber: g

Carbs: g

Protein: g

57. Iced Orange Punch

Preparation time: 10 minutes

Cooking time: 0

Servings: 8

Ingredients:

Ice Mold

Club soda

1 lemon, sliced

1 lime, sliced

Punch

1 quart each chilled orange juice (no sugar added), club soda, and diet ginger ale

Directions:

To Prepare Ice Mold: Pour enough club soda into a 10- or 12-cup ring mold to fill mold;

add lemon and lime slices, arranging them in an alternating pattern. Cover the mold and carefully transfer to freezer, freeze until solid. To Prepare Punch: In a large punch bowl, combine juice and sodas. Remove ice mold from ring mold and float ice mold in a punch.

Nutrition:

56 calories.

1 g protein.

0.1 g fat.

14 g carbohydrate.

35 mg sodium.

0 mg cholesterol

Chapter 11:

Desserts

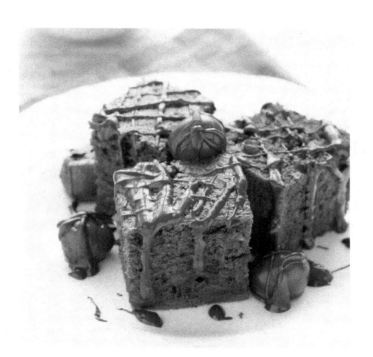

58. Chocolate Mousse

Preparation time: 6 mins

Cooking Time: 0 mins

Servings: 6

Ingredients:

16 ounces (2 cups) cream cheese

3-6 tablespoons of the desired sweetener

1/2 cup unsweetened cocoa powder

1/2 cup heavy whipped cream

One large avocado

90% dark chocolate, to garnish

1/4 teaspoon vanilla extract

Directions:

Beat cream cheese until it becomes smooth and creamy, slowly mix cocoa powder.

Add avocado and beat it nicely for 5 minutes until it becomes creamy.

Add vanilla and sweetener, and then hit it again until it becomes creamy and smooth. Place the whipped cream in the chocolate mixture and fold gently. Place the chocolate mousse in the desired containers. Garnish with dark chocolate chips.

Nutrition:

Calories: 333 Cal

Fat: 35 g Fiber: g

Carbs: 2 g Protein: 1 g

59. Chocolate Chia Pudding with Almonds

Preparation time: 10 mins

Cooking Time: 0 mins

Servings: 2

Ingredients:

Four tablespoons of chopped almonds

1 cup of water

Sweetener

½ cup heavy cream

Two tablespoons of cocoa powder

Six tablespoons of chia seeds

Two tablespoons of MCT oil

Directions:

Add chia seeds, heavy cream, water, MCT oil, cocoa powder, and sweetener in a bowl.

Mix them. Allow sitting for 7-11 hours. After 11 hours, add almonds. Your dish is ready.

Nutrition:

Calories: 288 Cal

Fat: 28 g Fiber: 8 g Carbs: 3 g

Protein: 4 g

60. Coconut Macadamia Chia Pudding

Preparation time: 10 mins

Cooking Time: 0 mins

Servings: 3

Ingredients:

Four tablespoons of macadamia nuts (chopped)

1 cup of water

Sweetener

½ cup coconut cream

Two tablespoons of MCT oil

Six tablespoons of chia seeds

Directions:

Add chia seeds, coconut cream, water, MCT oil and sweetener in a bowl. Mix them. Allow sitting for 7-11 hours, after 11 hours add macadamia nuts. Your dish is ready.

Nutrition:

Calories: 260 Cal Fat: 9 g

Fiber: 2 g Carbs: 2 g Protein: 2 g

61. Keto Chocolate Mug

Preparation time: 7 mins

Cooking Time: 0 mins

Servings: 1

Ingredients:

Two tablespoons of butter

One teaspoon sweetener

1/4 cup almond powder

1/2 teaspoon baking powder

Two tablespoons of cocoa powder

Pinch of salt

One big beaten egg

1/4 cup whipped cream, to serve

Two tablespoons of Keto-based chocolate chips

Directions:

Place the butter in a microwaveable cup and heat until melted for 30 seconds. Add remaining ingredients except for whipped cream and stir well. Microwave for 45 seconds to 1 minute, or until the cake set, but still fudgy. Serve with cream.

Nutrition:

Calories: 500 al

Fat: 50 g Fiber 3 g

Carbs: 2 g Protein: 7 g

62. Vanilla Chia Pudding

Preparation time: 5 mins

Cooking Time: 0 mins

Servings: 1

Ingredients:

Ingredients

1/2 cup strawberries

2 cups of water

Sweetener

½ cup heavy cream

Vanilla extract (few drops)

½ cup chia seeds

Two tablespoons MCT oil

Directions:

Add chia seeds, heavy cream, water, MCT oil, vanilla extract, and sweetener in a bowl. Mix them. Allow sitting for 7-11 hours. After 11 hours, add strawberries. Your dish is ready.

Nutrition: Calories: 550 Cal Fat: 57 g
Fiber: 3 g Carbs: 12 g Protein: 2 g

63. Choco Lava Cake

Preparation time: 20 mins

Cooking Time: 0 mins

Servings: 4

Ingredients:

2.5 ounces of dark chocolate

One tablespoon almond flour

1/4 cup coconut oil

1/4 teaspoon Vanilla extract

Two eggs

Cocoa powder for garnish

Two tablespoons of sweetener

Directions:

Preheat oven to 375 ° C. Grease two molds with coconut oil and sprinkle them with cocoa powder. Melt chocolate, coconut oil and add vanilla to it. Beat eggs and sweetener together in a different bowl.

Slowly add the chocolate mixture with egg mixture and beat until well mixed. Add the almond flour and mix until incorporated. Fill the molds evenly with the dough—Bake for 10 minutes. Serve immediately.

Nutrition:

Calories: 247 Cal

Fat: 24 g Fiber: 0 g

Carbs: 2 g Protein: 3 g

64. Coconut Cup Cakes

Preparation time: 35 mins

Cooking Time: 0 mins

Servings: 6

Ingredients:

Six tablespoons of coconut flour

1/2 cup hot water

1/2 cup unsalted coconut butter

One teaspoon vanilla extract

One tablespoon flaxseed

One teaspoon baking powder

Four tablespoons of stevia

Pinch of salt

For icing:

1 cup of raw cashews

Two tablespoons of Swerve

1/2 cup whole coconut milk

One teaspoon vanilla extract

Directions:

CUPCAKES:

Preheat oven to 350F. Grease 6 cupcake molds. Pour the water over the coconut butter and mix well, then add flaxseed, vanilla, stevia, and salt. Leave the flaxseed for few minutes to stow everything. In another bowl, combine baking powder and coconut flour.

Add flour mixture and flaxseed mixture slowly and stir until no lumps are left, and everything is smooth. Spread them in molds and bake for 20 to 25 minutes until the top is solid and the edges turn golden. Take them out of the oven and wait a few minutes for them to cool

FOR ICING:

Put all ingredients in a blender and blend for about 2-3 minutes until smooth. Add them to cupcakes. Sprinkle with dried coconut if you want

Nutrition:

Calories: 258 Cal

Fat: 25 g

Carbs: 3 g

Protein: 4 g

65. Easy Chocolate Cheesecake

Preparation time: 30 mins

Cooking Time: 0 mins

Servings: 4

Ingredients:

Two 1/2tablespoons of sour cream

Three tablespoons of erythritol powder

Five tablespoons of cream cheese

Three tablespoons of cocoa powder

Two tablespoons of butter

1/2 teaspoon vanilla extract

Crust

Two tablespoons of almond flour

Pinch of kosher salt

Two teaspoons of cocoa powder

Two teaspoons of butter

Two teaspoons of powdered erythritol

Directions:

Crust

Roast almond flour in a pan over medium heat until golden for 3 minutes. Pour the roasted almond flour into a small bowl and mix cocoa, sweetener, and salt. Add the butter and mix well. Press into a pastry mold or a plate and refrigerate while the cheesecake prepared.

Cake

Put the sour cream in a medium bowl and beat with an electric mixer for 3 minutes. Add cream cheese, butter, and beat with an electric mixer until the cream is thoroughly mixed. Add vanilla extract, sweetener, cocoa and beat until everything is mixed together.

Pour the mixture into the mold. Freeze for 20 to 30 minutes

Nutrition:

Calories: 200 Cal

Fat: 20 g

Carbs: 2 g

Protein: 2 g

66. Chocolate Chip Brownie

Preparation time: 43 mins

Cooking Time: 0 mins

Servings: 4

Ingredients:

1/2 cup MCT oil

Two teaspoons of erythritol

1/2 cup water 1/4 teaspoon baking powder

One teaspoon Vanilla extract

1/4 teaspoon salt 1/2 cup coconut flour

Keto Chocolate chips

Two tablespoons of cocoa powder

Directions:

ICING: Mix 1 tablespoon of cocoa powder and one tablespoon of MCT oil, mix well. Add a few drops of Vanilla extract, sweetener and mix them well.

BROWNIES: Preheat oven to 350 F. Put MCT oil, water, vanilla extract, coconut flour, chocolate chips, salt, baking powder and sweetener in a bowl and mix them all well. Let it cool for at least 10 minutes before baking.

Cover pan with parchment paper. Stir all mixture in the pan—Bake for 15 minutes. Allow the brownies to cool for 10 minutes before slicing and serving.

Nutrition: Calories: 300 Cal Fat: 29 g

Carbs: 2 g Protein: 2 g

67. Coconut Cookies

Preparation time: 37 mins

Cooking Time: 0 mins

Servings: 20

Ingredients:

3 cups of unsweetened coconut flakes

1/2 cup sugar-free maple syrup

1 cup of coconut oil

Directions:

Layout a large plate or baking tray with parchment paper and set aside. In a large bowl mix all ingredients and mix well.

Lightly moisten the hands, then form small balls with the dough and place them on the baking tray at a distance of 1 to 2 inches.

Tap on each biscuit with a fork.

Cool until firm.

Nutrition:

Calories: 90 Cal

Fat: 9 g

Carbs: 0.5 g

Protein: 0 g

68. Choco Pie

Preparation time: 50 mins

Cooking Time: 0 mins

Servings: 6

Ingredients:

Filling

 Crust

½ cup dark chocolate

 2 1/2 tablespoons of water

Two teaspoons of stevia powder

three tablespoons of coconut oil

2 cups of coconut milk cream

one teaspoon stevia powder

One tablespoon coconut water

one tablespoon flaxseed

1 1/2 cups of crushed hazelnuts

1 1/2 cups of almond flour

Pinch of salt

One teaspoon vanilla extract

Directions:

Crust

Preheat oven to 350 F. Covers the baking pan with parchment sheet. Stir the dry ingredients together in a bowl and mix them well. Combine the flax seeds and water in another small bowl and set aside. Let the seeds get thick. Pour the flax mixture and the melted coconut oil over the dry ingredients and mix well.

Firmly press the dough into the mold base. Use a fork to prick the crust. Bake the crust for about 15 minutes until its firm and slightly browned. Set aside to let it cool.

Filing

Put roasted hazelnuts in a blender, blend until oil is released and liquid state obtained. Add melted chocolate and salt. Put the coconut cream in another bowl. Add vanilla, one tablespoon of Coconut water and sweetener. Beat the cream with the hand blender for 60 seconds or more until it gets soft and fluffy. Carefully stir the cream with the chocolate mixture. Taste it and add some sweetener if needed. Pour the filling over the crust. Freeze for 2 hours until the mix is ready.

Nutrition:

Calories: 300 Cal

Fat: 28 g

Carbs: 3 g

Protein: 1 g

69. Keto Blueberry Muffins

Preparation time: 40 mins

Cooking Time: 0 mins

Servings: 6

Ingredients:

1 Stick/ ½ cup/113 grams butter

One teaspoon vanilla

Eight tablespoons of fresh cheese

Dry ingredients

1 cup of coconut fibers

1/4 teaspoon Xanthan chewing gum

Two teaspoons of baking soda

1/8 teaspoon cinnamon

1/2 teaspoon salt

Wet Ingredients

Six medium eggs

1/2 cup heavy cream

And the Last

¾ cup blueberries

Four teaspoons of coffee

Directions:

Mix butter, vanilla and cream cheese in a bowl add two eggs and beat the mixture again. Now add 1/3rd of the dry ingredients and mix properly. Add two more eggs and half of the dry ingredients and beat the mixture again. Now add last two eggs and remaining of the dry ingredients and mix them properly. Finish the mixture by adding heavy cream and mix it properly until fully incorporated.

Add the berries and mix again. Now fill them in muffin containers and bake them for 30 minutes at 400 degrees F. Your muffins are ready.

Nutrition:

Calories: 214 Cal Fat: 19 g

Carbs: 6 g Protein: 6 g

70. Keto Oven-Baked Brie Cheese

Preparation time: 30 mins

Cooking Time: 0 mins

Servings: 8

Ingredients:

2 cups brie or Camembert cheese

One tablespoon olive oil

15 pecans or walnuts

Salt and pepper

One garlic clove

One tablespoon fresh rosemary

Directions:

Preheat the oven to 400 ° F (200 ° C). Place the cheese on a baking tray lined with baking paper or in a small non-stick pan. Chop the garlic and roughly chop the nuts and herbs. Mix the three with olive oil. Add salt and pepper.

Put the walnut mixture over the cheese and bake for 10 minutes or until the cheese is lukewarm and soft and the nuts are toasted. Serve warm or tepid.

Nutrition:

Calories: 231 Cal

Fat: 23 g

Carbs: 4 g

Protein: 2 g

71. Keto Vanilla Pound Cake

Preparation time: 1hr 5 mins

Cooking Time: 0 mins

Servings: 8

Ingredients:

2 cups of almond flour

One teaspoon of vanilla extract

1/2 cup butter

1 cup sour cream

1 cup erythritol

2 ounces / 4 tablespoon of cream cheese

Two teaspoons of baking powder

Four big eggs

Directions:

Preheat the oven to 350 degrees Fahrenheit.

Butter generously to a 9-inch pan set aside.

Combine almond flour and baking powder in a large bowl, set aside. Cut the butter into several small squares and place in a separate bowl, add the cream cheese.

Microwave butter and cream cheese for 30 seconds. Be careful not to burn the cream cheese. Mix these ingredients until well combined. Add erythritol, vanilla extract and sour cream to the butter and cream cheese mixture. Mix well.

Pour the wet ingredients into a large bowl of almond flour and baking soda. Mix well. Add the eggs to the dough. Mix well. Place the money in the buttered pan and bake for 50 minutes.

For best results, allow the cake to cool completely for at least 2 hours, preferably overnight. If you remove it too soon, it may collapse a bit.

Nutrition:

Calories: 330 Cal

Fat: 32 g

Carbs: 2 g

Protein: 4 g

Chapter 12:

Snacks

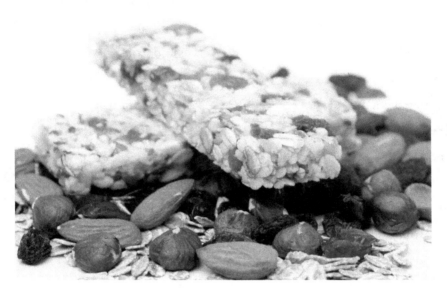

72. Superfoods Raw Vegan Cookies

Preparation time: 10 mins

Cooking Time: 30 mins

Servings: 4

Ingredients:

½ cup of coconut milk

½ cup of cocoa powder

½ cup of coconut oil ½ cup raw honey

2 cups finely shredded coconut

1 cup large flake coconut

2 tsp of ground vanilla bean

½ cup chopped almonds or chia seeds (optional) ½ cup almond butter (optional)

Directions:

Combine the coconut milk, cocoa powder, and coconut oil in a saucepan. I think that it still counts as a raw dessert if you have to warm up the coconut milk and coconut oil.

So, warm up the mixture over medium heat because we want the coconut oil to melt and become liquid.

Nutrition: Calories: 212 Cal Fat: 14 g

Carbs: 20 g Protein: 4 g

73. Raw Vegan Walnuts Pie Crust and Fresh Brownies

Preparation time: 10 mins

Cooking Time: 30 mins

Servings: 4

Ingredients:

1½ cups walnuts 1 cup pitted dates

1½ tsp ground vanilla bean

2 tsp chia seeds

1/3 cup unsweetened cocoa powder

Topping for raw brownies:

1/3 cup almond butter

Directions:

Add walnuts to a food processor or blender. Mix until finely ground.

Add the vanilla, dates, and cocoa powder to the blender.

Mix well and optionally add a couple of drops of water at a time to make the mixture stick together.

That is an essential raw walnuts pie crust recipe.

You can use almonds or cashews as well.

If you need a pie crust, then spread it thinly in a 9-inch disc and add the filling.

If you want to make raw brownies, then transfer the mixture into a small dish and top with almond butter.

Nutrition: Calories: 320 Cal Fat: 32 g Carbs: 6 g Protein: 10 g

74. Raw Vegan Reese's Cups

Preparation time: 10 mins

Cooking Time: 35 mins

Servings: 4

Ingredients:

"Peanut" butter filling

½ cup sunflower seeds butter

½ cup almond butter

1 tbsp raw honey

2 tbsp melted coconut oil

Superfoods chocolate part:

½ cup cacao powder

2 tbsp raw honey

1/3 cup of coconut oil (melted)

Directions:

Mix the "peanut" butter filling ingredients.

Put a spoonful of the mixture into each muffin cup.

Refrigerate.

Mix superfoods chocolate ingredients.

Put a spoonful of the superfood's chocolate mixture over the "peanut" butter mixture. Freeze!

Nutrition: Calories: 320 Cal Fat: 32 g Carbs: 6 g Protein: 10 g

75. Raw Vegan Coffee Cashew Cream Cake

Preparation time: 10 mins

Cooking Time: 35 mins

Servings: 4

Ingredients:

Coffee cashew cream

2 cups raw cashews

1 tsp of ground vanilla bean

3 tbsp melted coconut oil

¼ cup raw honey

1/3 cup solid coffee or triple espresso shot

Directions:

Blend all ingredients for the cream, pour it onto the crust and refrigerate.

Garnish with coffee beans.

Nutrition:

Calories: 80 Cal

Fat: 5 g

Carbs: 6 g

Protein: 2 g

76. Raw Vegan Chocolate Cashew Truffles

Preparation time: 10 mins

Cooking Time: 35 mins

Servings: 4

Ingredients:

1 cup ground cashews

1 tsp of ground vanilla bean

½ cup of coconut oil

¼ cup raw honey

2 tbsp flax meal

2 tbsp hemp hearts

2 tbsp cacao powder

Directions:

Mix all ingredients and make truffles. Sprinkle coconut flakes on top.

Nutrition:

Calories: 65 Cal

Fat: 5 g

Carbs: 3 g

Protein: 1 g

77. Raw Vegan Double Almond Raw Chocolate Tart

Preparation time: 10 mins

Cooking Time: 35 mins

Servings: 4

Ingredients:

1½ cups of raw almonds

¼ cup of coconut oil, melted

1 tbsp raw honey or royal jelly

8 ounces dark chocolate, chopped

1 cup of coconut milk

½ cup unsweetened shredded coconut

Directions:

Crust:

Ground almonds and add melted coconut oil, raw honey and combine.

Using a spatula, spread this mixture into the tart or pie pan.

Filling:

Put the chopped chocolate in a bowl, heat coconut milk and pour over chocolate and whisk together.

Pour filling into tart shell.

Refrigerate.

Toast almond slivers chips and sprinkle over tart.

Nutrition: Calories: 139 Cal Fat: 10 g Carbs: 9 g Protein: 0 g

78. Raw Vegan Bounty Bars

Preparation time: 10 mins

Cooking Time: 35 mins

Servings: 4

Ingredients:

"Peanut" butter filling

2 cups desiccated coconut

3 tbsp coconut oil - melted

1 cup of coconut cream - full fat

4 tbsp of raw honey

1 tsp ground vanilla bean

Pinch of sea salt

Superfoods chocolate part:

½ cup cacao powder

2 tbsp raw honey

1/3 cup of coconut oil (melted)

Directions:

Mix the coconut oil, coconut cream, honey, vanilla, and salt. Pour over desiccated coconut and mix well. Mold the coconut mixture into balls, small bars similar to bounty and freeze.

Or pour the whole mixture into a tray, freeze and cut into small bars.

Make superfoods chocolate mixture, warm it up and dip frozen coconut into the chocolate and put on a tray and freeze again.

Nutrition: Calories: 68 Cal Fat: 2 g Carbs: 9 g Protein: 1 g

79. Raw Vegan Tartlets with Coconut Cream

Preparation time: 10 mins

Cooking Time: 35 mins

Servings: 4

Ingredients:

Pudding:

One avocado

2 tbsp coconut oil

2 tbsp raw honey

2 tbsp cacao powder

1 tsp ground vanilla bean

Pinch of salt

¼ cup almond milk, as needed

Add ½ tsp cinnamon and whip again.

Directions:

Blend all the ingredients in the food processor until smooth and thick.

Spread evenly into tartlet crusts.

Optionally, put some goji berries on top of the pudding layer.

Make the coconut cream, spread it on top of the pudding layer, and put back in the fridge overnight.

Serve with one blueberry on top of each tartlet.

Nutrition: Calories: 87 Cal Fat: 9 g

Carbs: 1 g Protein: 1 g

80. Raw Vegan "Peanut" Butter Truffles

Preparation time: 10 mins

Cooking Time: 30 mins

Servings: 4

Ingredients:

5 tbsp sunflower seed butter

1 tbsp coconut oil

1 tbsp raw honey

1 tsp ground vanilla bean

¾ cup almond flour

1 tbsp flaxseed meal

Pinch of salt

1 tbsp cacao butter

hemp hearts (optional)

¼ cup superfoods chocolate

Directions:

Mix until all ingredients are incorporated.

Roll the dough into 1-inch balls, place them on parchment paper and refrigerate for half an hour (yield about 14 truffles).

Dip each truffle in the melted superfoods chocolate, one at the time.

Place them back on the pan with parchment paper or coat them in cocoa powder or coconut flakes.

Nutrition: Calories: 73 Cal Fat: 5 g

Carbs: 7 g Protein: 0 g

81. Raw Vegan Chocolate Pie

Preparation time: 10 mins

Cooking Time: 25 mins

Servings: 4

Ingredients:

Crust:

2 cups almonds, soaked overnight and drained

1 cup pitted dates, soaked overnight and drained

1 cup chopped dried apricots

1½ tsp ground vanilla bean

2 tsp chia seeds

One banana

Filling:

4 tbsp raw cacao powder

3 tbsp raw honey

Two ripe avocados

2 tbsp organic coconut oil

2 tbsp almond milk (if needed, check for consistency first)

Directions:

Add almonds and banana to a food processor or blender.

Mix until it forms a thick ball.

Add the vanilla, dates, and apricot chunks to the blender.

Mix well and optionally add a couple of drops of water at a time to make the mixture stick together.

Spread in a 10-inch dis.

Mix filling ingredients in a blender and add almond milk if necessary.

Add filling to the crust and refrigerate.

Nutrition:

Calories: 278 Cal Fat: 21 g Carbs: 19 g

Protein: 0 g

82. Raw Vegan Chocolate Walnut Truffles

Preparation time: 10 mins

Cooking Time: 35 mins

Servings: 4

Ingredients:

1 cup ground walnuts

1 tsp cinnamon

½ cup of coconut oil

¼ cup raw honey

2 tbsp chia seeds

2 tbsp cacao powder

Directions:

Mix all ingredients and make truffles.

Coat with cinnamon, coconut flakes or chopped almonds.

Nutrition: Calories: 130 Cal Fat: 11 g

Carbs: 6 g Protein: 2 g

83. Raw Vegan Carrot Cake

Preparation time: 10 mins

Cooking Time: 35 mins

Servings: 4

Ingredients:

Crust:

Four carrots, chopped

1½ cups oats

½ cup dried coconut

2 cups dates

1 tsp cinnamon

½ tsp nutmeg

1½ cups cashews

2 tbsp coconut oil

Juice from 1 lemon

2 tbsp raw honey

1 tsp ground vanilla bean

Water, as needed

Directions:

Add all crust ingredients to the blender.

Mix well and optionally add a couple of drops of water at a time to make the mixture stick together.

Press in a small pan.

Take it out and put on a plate and freeze.

Mix frosting ingredients in a blender and add water if necessary.

Add frosting to the crust and refrigerate.

Nutrition:

Calories: 60 Cal

Fat: 3 g

Carbs: 10 g

Protein: 1 g

84. Frozen Raw Blackberry Cake

Preparation time: 10 mins

Cooking Time: 45 mins

Servings: 4

Ingredients:

Crust:

3⁄4 cup shredded coconut

15 dried dates soaked in hot water and drained

1/3 cup pumpkin seeds

1⁄4 cup of coconut oil

Middle filling

Coconut whipped cream - see Coconut Whipped Cream recipes.

Top filling:

1 pound of frozen blackberries

3-4 tbsp raw honey

1⁄4 cup of coconut cream

Two egg whites

Directions:

Grease the cake tin with coconut oil and mix all base ingredients in the blender until you get a sticky ball.

Press the base mixture in a cake tin.

Freeze.

Make Coconut Whipped Cream.

Process berries and add honey, coconut cream and egg whites.

Pour middle filling - Coconut Whipped Cream in the tin and spread evenly.

Freeze.

Pour top filling - berries mixture-in the tin, spread, decorate with blueberries and almonds, and return to freezer.

Nutrition:

Calories: 12 Cal Fat: 0 g

Carbs: 3 g Protein: 0 g

85. Raw Vegan Chocolate Hazelnuts Truffles

Preparation time: 10 mins

Cooking Time: 30 mins

Servings: 4

Ingredients:

1 cup ground almonds

1 tsp ground vanilla bean

½ cup of coconut oil

½ cup mashed pitted dates

12 whole hazelnuts

2 tbsp cacao powder

Directions:

Mix all ingredients and make truffles with one whole hazelnut in the middle.

Nutrition: Calories: 35 Cal Fat: 3 g Carbs: 1 g Protein: 1 g

86. Raw Vegan Chocolate Cream Fruity Cake

Preparation time: 10 mins

Cooking Time: 45 mins

Servings: 4

Ingredients:

One avocado 2 tbsp raw honey

2 tbsp coconut oil 2 tbsp cacao powder

1 tsp ground vanilla bean

Pinch of sea salt

¼ cup of coconut milk

1 tbsp coconut flakes

Fruits:

One chopped banana 1 cup pitted cherries.

Directions:

Prepare the crust and press it at the bottom of the pan. Blend all chocolate cream ingredients, fold in the fruits, and pour in the crust. Whip the top layer, spread, and sprinkle with cacao powder. Refrigerate.

Nutrition: Calories: 68 Cal Fat: 3 g

Carbs: 9 g Protein: 0 g

Chapter 13:
Dressings

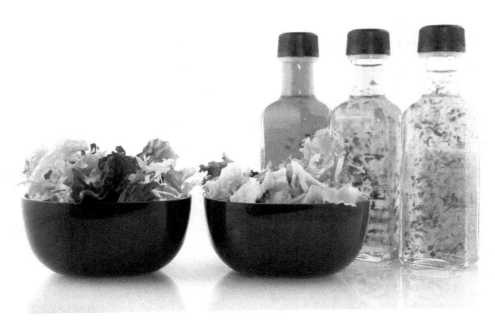

87. Vinaigrette

Preparation time: 5 mins

Cooking Time: 0 mins

Servings: 1

Ingredients:

4 teaspoons Mustard yellow

4 tablespoon White wine vinegar

1 teaspoon Honey

5.6 oz Olive oil

Directions:

Whisk the mustard, vinegar, and honey in a bowl with a whisk until they are well mixed.

Add the olive oil in small amounts while whisking with a whisk until the vinaigrette is thick.

SEASON WITH SALT AND PEPPER.

Nutrition: Calories: 80 Cal Fat: 9 g

Carbs: 1 g Protein: 0 g

88. Spicy Ras-el-Han Out Dressing

Preparation time: 11 mins

Cooking Time: 0 mins

Servings: 1

Ingredients:

4.2 oz Olive oil

1-piece Lemon (the juice)

2 teaspoons Honey

1 ½ teaspoon Ras el Han out

1⁄2 pieces Red pepper

Directions:

Remove the seeds from the chili pepper.

Chop the chili pepper as finely as possible.

Place the pepper in a bowl with lemon juice, honey, and Ras-El-Han out and whisk with a whisk.

THEN ADD THE OLIVE OIL DROP BY DROP WHILE CONTINUING TO WHISK.

Nutrition:

Calories: 15 Cal Fat: 0 g Carbs: 1 g

Protein: 0 g

89. Mustard

Preparation time: 15 mins

Cooking Time: 0 mins

Servings: 1

Ingredients:

0.13 lb Mustard seeds

1/4 cup Water

4 tablespoon Apple cider vinegar

2 teaspoons Lemon juice

0.2 lb Honey

1⁄2 teaspoon dried turmeric

Directions:

Put mustard seeds, water, and vinegar in a glass, close well and leave in the fridge for 12 hours.

Put all ingredients in a tall measuring cup the next day.

Use your hand blender to puree everything.

Try the mustard and add some honey or salt.

STORE THE MUSTARD IN A CLEAN GLASS IN THE FRIDGE, IT WILL KEEP FOR AT LEAST 3 WEEKS.

Nutrition:

Calories: 60 Cal

Fat: 3 g

Carbs: 5 g

Protein: 3 g

90. Cucumber Salad with Lime and Coriander

Preparation time: 20 mins

Cooking Time: 0 mins

Servings: 1

Ingredients:

1-piece Red onion

2 pieces Cucumber

2 pieces Lime (juice)

2 tablespoon fresh coriander

Directions:

Cut the onion into rings and thinly slice the cucumber. Chop the coriander finely.

Place the onion rings in a bowl and season with about half a tablespoon of salt.

Rub it in well and then fill the bowl with water.

Pour off the water and then rinse the onion rings thoroughly (in a sieve).

Put the cucumber slices together with onion, lime juice, coriander and olive oil in a salad bowl and stir everything well.

Season with a little salt.

YOU CAN KEEP THIS DISH IN THE REFRIGERATOR IN A COVERED BOWL FOR A FEW DAYS.

Nutrition: Calories: 168 Cal Fat: 3 g

Carbs: 29 g Protein: 3 g

91. Honey Mustard Dressing

Preparation time: 15 mins

Cooking Time: 0 mins

Servings: 1

Ingredients:

4 tablespoon Olive oil

11/2 teaspoon Honey

11/2 teaspoon Mustard

1 teaspoon Lemon juice

1 pinch Salt

Directions:

Mix olive oil, honey, mustard, and lemon juice into an even dressing with a whisk.

SEASON WITH SALT.

Nutrition:

Calories: 150 Cal

Fat: 12 g

Carbs: 0 g

Protein: 0 g

92. Caesar Dressing

Preparation time: 10 mins

Cooking Time: 0 mins

Servings: 1

Ingredients:

8.4 oz Olive oil

2 tablespoons Lemon juice

4 pieces Anchovy fillet

2 tablespoon Mustard yellow

1 clove Garlic

1/2 teaspoon Salt

1/2 teaspoon Black pepper

Directions:

Remove the peel from the garlic and chop it finely.

Put all ingredients in a blender and puree evenly.

THIS DRESSING CAN BE KEPT IN THE FRIDGE FOR ABOUT 3 DAYS.

Nutrition:

Calories: 90 Cal

Fat: 9 g

Carbs: 0 g

Protein: 0 g

93. Basil Dressing

Preparation time: 5 mins

Cooking Time: 0 mins

Servings: 1

Ingredients:

Fresh basil 0.22 lb

Shallots 1 piece

Garlic 1 clove

Olive oil (mild) 4.2 oz

White wine vinegar 2 tablespoon

Directions:

Finely chop the shallot and garlic.

Put the shallot, garlic, basil, olive oil and vinegar in a blender.

Mix it into an even mix.

Season the dressing and season with salt and pepper.

PLACE THE DRESSING IN A CLEAN GLASS AND STORE IN THE REFRIGERATOR. IT STAYS FRESH AND TASTY FOR AT LEAST 3 DAYS.

Nutrition:

Calories: 45 Cal

Fat: 4 g

Carbs: 1 g

Protein: 0 g

94. Fresh Chicory Salad

Preparation time: 10 mins

Cooking Time: 0 mins

Servings: 1

Ingredients:

1-piece Orange

1-piece Tomato

1/4 pieces Cucumber

1/4 pieces Red onion

Directions:

Cut off the hard stem of the chicory and remove the leaves.

Peel the orange and cut the pulp into wedges.

Cut the tomatoes and cucumbers into small pieces.

Cut the red onion into thin half rings.

Place the chicory boats on a plate, spread the orange wedges, tomato, cucumber and red onion over the boats.

DRIZZLE SOME OLIVE OIL AND FRESH LEMON JUICE ON THE DISH.

Nutrition:

Calories: 112 Cal

Fat: 11 g

Carbs: 2 g

Protein: 0 g

95. Steak Salad

Preparation time: 30 mins

Cooking Time: 0 mins

Servings: 1

Ingredients:

2 pieces Beef steak

2 cloves Garlic

1-piece Red onion

2 pieces Egg

1 hand Cherry tomatoes

2 hands Lettuce

1-piece Avocado

1/2 pieces Cucumber

1 pinch Season white Salt

1 pinch Black pepper

Directions:

Place the steaks in a flat bowl. Pour the olive oil over the steaks and press the garlic over it. Turn the steaks a few times so that they are covered with oil and garlic. Cover the meat and let it marinate for at least 1 hour. Boil eggs. Heat a grill pan and fry the steaks medium. Take the steaks out of the pan, wrap them in aluminum foil and let them rest for 5 to 10 minutes. Spread the lettuce on the plates. Cut the steaks into slices and place them in the middle of the salad. Cut the eggs into wedges, the cucumber into half-moons, the red onion into thin half-rings, the cherry tomatoes into halves and the avocado into slices. Spread this around the steaks.

Drizzle over the olive oil and white wine vinegar and season with a little salt and pepper.

Calories: 102 Cal

Fat: 3 g

Carbs: 0 g

Protein: 9 g

96. Zucchini Salad with Lemon Chicken

Preparation time: 40 mins

Cooking Time: 0 mins

Servings: 2

Ingredients:

1-piece Zucchini

1-piece yellow zucchini

1 hand Cherry tomatoes

2 pieces Chicken breast

1-piece Lemon

2 tablespoons Olive oil

Directions:

Use a meat mallet or a heavy pan to make the chicken fillets as thin as possible.

Put the fillets in a bowl.

Squeeze the lemon over the chicken and add the olive oil. Cover it and let it marinate for at least 1 hour.

Heat a pan over medium-high heat and fry the chicken until cooked through and browned. Season with salt and pepper.

Make zucchini from the zucchini and put in a bowl.

Quarter the tomatoes and stir in the zucchini.

Slice the chicken fillets diagonally and place them on the salad. Drizzle the salad with a little olive oil and season with salt and pepper.

Nutrition: Calories: 170 Cal Fat: 5 g

Carbs: 25 g Protein: 6 g

97. Fresh Salad with Orange Dressing

Preparation time: 10 mins

Cooking Time: 0 mins

Servings: 2

Ingredients:

1 / 2 fruit Salad 1-piece yellow bell pepper

1-piece Red pepper 0.22 lb Carrot (grated)

1 hand Almonds

Ingredients dressing:

4 tablespoon Olive oil

3.7 oz Orange juice (fresh)

1 tablespoon Apple cider vinegar

Directions:

Clean the peppers and cut them into long thin strips.

Tear off the lettuce leaves and cut them into smaller pieces.

Mix the salad with the peppers and the carrots processed with the Julienne peeler in a bowl.

Roughly chop the almonds and sprinkle over the salad.

Mix all the ingredients for the dressing in a bowl.

POUR THE DRESSING OVER THE SALAD JUST BEFORE SERVING.

Nutrition:

Calories: 45 Cal Fat: 3 g

Carbs: 4 g Protein: 0 g

98. Tomato and Avocado Salad

Preparation time: 15 mins

Cooking Time: 0 mins

Servings: 3

Ingredients:

1-piece Tomato 1-piece Cherry tomatoes

1 / 2 pieces Red onion

1-piece Avocado

Taste fresh oregano

1 1 / 2 cup Olive oil

1 teaspoon White wine vinegar

1 teaspoon Celtic sea salt

Directions:

Cut the tomato into thick slices.

Cut half of the cherry tomatoes into slices and the other half in half.

Cut the red onion into super thin half rings. (or use a mandolin for this)

Cut the avocado into 6 parts.

Spread the tomatoes on a plate, place the avocado on top and sprinkle the red onion over them. Sprinkle fresh oregano on the salad as desired.

DRIZZLE OLIVE OIL AND VINEGAR ON THE SALAD WITH A PINCH OF SALT.

Nutrition:Calories: 41 Cal Fat: 3 g Carbs: 1 g Protein: 1 g

99. Spinach Salad with Green Asparagus and Salmon

Preparation time: 12 mins

Cooking Time: 0 mins

Servings: 1

Ingredients:

0.44 lb Spinach

2 pieces Egg

0.26 lb smoked salmon

0.22 lb Asparagus tips

0.33 lb Cherry tomatoes

Lemon 1/2 pieces

1 teaspoon Olive oil

Directions:

Cook the eggs the way you like them.

Heat a pan with a little oil and fry the asparagus tips al dente.

Halve cherry tomatoes.

Place the spinach on a plate and spread the asparagus tips, cherry tomatoes and smoked salmon on top.

Scare, peel, and halve the eggs. Add them to the salad.

Squeeze the lemon over the lettuce and drizzle some olive oil over it.

Season the salad with a little salt and pepper.

Nutrition: Calories: 54 Cal Fat: 0 g

Carbs: 1 g Protein: 1 g

100.   Brunoised Salad

Preparation time: 16 mins

Cooking Time: 0 mins

Servings: 1

Ingredients:

1-piece Meat tomato

1/2 pieces Zucchini

1/2 pieces Red bell pepper

1/2 pieces yellow bell pepper

1/2 pieces Red onion

3 sprigs fresh parsley

1/4 pieces Lemon

2 tablespoons Olive oil

Directions:

Finely dice the tomatoes, zucchini, peppers, and red onions to get a brunoised.

Mix all the cubes in a bowl.

Chop parsley and mix in the salad.

Squeeze the lemon over the salad and add the olive oil.

SEASON WITH SALT AND PEPPER.

Nutrition:

Calories: 42 Cal

Fat: 2 g

Carbs: 3 g

Protein: 0 g

101. Broccoli Salad

Preparation time: 30 mins

Cooking Time: 0 mins

Servings: 1

Ingredients:

1-piece Broccoli

1/2 pieces Red onion

0.22 lb Carrot (grated)

0.22 lb Red grapes

Ingredients dressing:

2 1/2 tablespoon Coconut yogurts

1 tablespoon Water

1 teaspoon Mustard yellow

1 teaspoon Salt

Directions:

Cut the broccoli into small florets and cook al dente for 5 minutes.

Cut the red onion into thin half rings.

Halve the grapes.

Mix coconut yogurt, water, and mustard with a pinch of salt to make an even dressing.

Drain the broccoli and rinse with ice-cold water to stop the cooking process.

Mix the broccoli with the carrot, onion, and red grapes in a bowl.

SERVE THE DRESSING SEPARATELY ON THE SIDE.

Nutrition:

Calories: 57 Cal

Fat: 4 g

Carbs: 8 g

Protein: 2 g

Conclusion

The fantastic world of Sirtuins that we have only begun to explore with this book, still reserves some great surprises and potential benefits for humankind and its biology and nutrition. There would still be much to write, as it is true, moreover, that still much remains to be studied and understood on these phenomenal enzymatic proteins.

First of all, however, we can already draw conclusions in this regard: taking foods rich in Sirtuin has significant benefits for our health, and it would seem, at the current state of research that there are no contraindications whatsoever. However, it remains essential to reiterate the importance of a varied, well-balanced diet and the absolute need for a medical-scientific opinion, before embarking on a change of diet, because we may have previous pathologies that could suffer an increase in change of diet.

It must also be said, as we have already done several times during the course of work, that a diet, however incredibly efficient it may seem on paper, and even magical, is not, in fact, a magic slimming elixir, but that as in any case of life, to get results it takes discipline, knowledge of the subject and perseverance.

Exercise remains something indispensable, both to lose weight, to stay fit and have a healthy life.

We therefore advise you to stop the diet immediately if you experience discomfort or situations that can endanger your own and / or someone else's health.

From the research conducted so far, another element that has a key role in this Sirt diet emerges, namely Resveratrol, a substance present in red wine and capable of acting as an activator for Sirtuins and their fat-burning mechanism. it is also good to note that a diet rich in Sirtuin and Resveratrol, in addition to burning fat, also manages to induce in the body the triggering of anti-aging and anti-oxidation of the cells, promoting cellular respiration, and therefore going to fight against dangerous free radicals, which are responsible for many human diseases.

THE SIRTFOOD DIET COOKBOOK

The latter condition can be mimicked by the daily intake of moderate quantities of red wine and foods rich in Sirtuins, such as those we mentioned in our book.

However, we are advising you to moderate wine consumption, as well as moderation in following this diet, because your health is the first thing we care about.

Because on the other hand, as Confucius said: "Moderation is the way to a long and happy life". Peace and prosperity to all of you.

A little piece of advice. If you want your body to be healthy and sexy, the only thing you will do is follow the steps on how the Sirtfood Diet works and to hold back your cravings especially to the food you used to eat. Because if you follow these steps of how the Sirtfood diet work but your body and mind want to eat the food you used to eat it is useless. So, change your mind set from the older you to the new you and do the Sirtfood diet.

CPSIA information can be obtained
at www.ICGtesting.com
Printed in the USA
LVHW101418211120
672149LV00009B/284